After The Before & After

A real-life story of weight loss,
weight gain
and weightlessness
through total acceptance

Published in the United States by Booklocker.com, Inc., Bangor, Maine.

Printed in the United States of America on acid-free paper.

KCLAnderson.com
2011

First Edition

DISCLAIMER

This book details the author's personal experiences with and opinions about weight loss, naturopathic medicine and hormone replacement therapy. The author is not a healthcare provider.

The author and publisher are providing this book and its contents on an "as is" basis and make no representations or warranties of any kind with respect to this book or its contents. The author and publisher disclaim all such representations and warranties, including for example warranties of merchantability and healthcare for a particular purpose. In addition, the author and publisher do not represent or warrant that the information accessible via this book is accurate, complete or current.

The statements made about products and services have not been evaluated by the U.S. Food and Drug Administration. They are not intended to diagnose, treat, cure, or prevent any condition or disease. Please consult with your own physician or healthcare specialist regarding the suggestions and recommendations made in this book.

Except as specifically stated in this book, neither the author or publisher, nor any authors, contributors, or other representatives will be liable for damages arising out of or in connection with the use of this book. This is a comprehensive limitation of liability that applies to all damages of any kind, including (without limitation) compensatory; direct, indirect or consequential damages; loss of data, income or profit; loss of or damage to property and claims of third parties.

You understand that this book is not intended as a substitute for consultation with a licensed healthcare practitioner, such as your physician. Before you begin any healthcare program, or change your lifestyle in any way, you will consult your physician or other licensed healthcare practitioner to ensure that you are in good health and that the examples contained in this book will not harm you.

This book provides content related to topics physical and/or mental health issues. As such, use of this book implies your acceptance of this disclaimer.

After The Before & After
A real-life story of weight loss, weight gain and weightlessness through total acceptance

Karen C.L. Anderson

This book is dedicated to every person
who ever lost weight and gained it back.

Table of Contents

About the Author

Karen C.L Anderson is a writer, speaker, blogger, communicator, right-brainer, ah-ha moment creator, and lover of what is.

She lives in Southeastern Connecticut with her husband Tim and their two cats, Bella and Starla.

For more information about her work, please visit www.kclanderson.com

*"If you can see your path laid out in front of you
step by step, you know it's not your path.
Your own path you make with every step you take.
That's why it's your path."*
~ Joseph Campbell

What This Book Is And What It Isn't

This book is about me, my reactions, and my memories. Others may remember certain situations that I recount in this book differently than I do. I am aware that others may have experienced some of the situations I write about in a way that was significantly different from the way I portray them here.

It is not a book about how to lose weight.

It is about my belief that if I could just accept myself, my body would respond in a positive way.

It's not a linear story or a memoir in the traditional sense, but rather a series of small evolutionary steps.

It's about realizing that it doesn't happen all at once…that it takes time and continued immersion and having to think about stuff more than once. It's about how you might know something, but that you might not "get it."

It's about working through the rough spots. It's about what it's like to take two steps forward and one step back, and then two steps back and one step forward, and how to be okay with that. And it's ultimately about realizing that there is no such thing as a step back.

It's about accepting yourself, no matter what. It's about realizing that it takes as long as it needs to take.

And that's okay.

The Back Story

"We nurture and care for the things
we love and feel connected to.
We neglect and destroy the things we do not." ~ Unknown

My story is both unique and universal.

I have been overweight or obese most of my adult life, and I have played at losing weight many times over the past 35 years. There were times when it really bothered me, and other times when it really didn't. I had a pretty good career. I traveled extensively. I had friends and boyfriends, and eventually, I married a wonderful man. I considered myself to be happy, smart, pretty, successful, loving, and lovable. Sometimes.

Deep down inside, however, my weight was an intensely emotional subject. It could bring me to tears in the doctor's office. If my mother brought it up, I'd get angry. Despite "happy, smart, pretty, successful, loving, and lovable," self-doubt and fear seemed to permeate my life.

For a long time, I stuffed those feelings down with food. Every once in a while, I would think about trying to lose weight, and perhaps, I'd make some sort of effort. I read books, tried various programs, and even took weight-loss drugs. I'd lose some weight, then gain it back...and more. In my head, I went back and forth between wanting to just accept and love myself the way I was, and wanting to just lose the damn weight already.

Then one day (in 2004), I noticed that a good friend had lost some weight. I asked what she was doing and she said she had joined a popular diet web site. I decided to join too.

But it didn't work.

I resisted following the food and exercise plans that were provided. That resistance combined with anger. I didn't want to follow a plan or count calories, I didn't want it to be hard, and I didn't want to try.

I could hear my mother's voice in my head: "You must not really want it. If you did, you'd go ahead and do it." She said that about everything. And she was right: I guess I didn't REALLY want to lose weight because if I did, then I'd just do it, right? I certainly knew how: eat right and exercise, calories in/calories out.

Obviously, I wasn't ready. So once again, I pushed those feelings away – the fear, the self-doubt, the resistance, the anger – and I quit.

But the realization that I didn't want to lose weight stayed with me. As 2004 came to a close, I took a deep breath and decided to try once again. In addition to the diet, however, I wanted to figure out the whys: Why don't I want to lose weight? Why do I want the easy way out? Why is it so hard? Why do I resist?

Instead of traditional counseling, I went to a hypnotherapist named Lynn Gaffin who specializes in Emotional Freedom Technique, or EFT. EFT combines two well-established sciences: mind-body medicine and acupuncture – without needles. It involves stimulating certain meridian points on the body. EFT practitioners tap on them with their fingertips as the patient recites a phrase or script that resonates with what the patient wants to achieve.

During the first session, it became clear what my problem was. Lynn asked me why I was there, and I poured out my whole sad, fat history. She started tapping with this phrase, which I was to repeat as she tapped: "Even though I am overweight, I love and accept myself."

The words stuck in my throat. I couldn't say it because I didn't believe it. I didn't love and accept myself. Instead, I sobbed. Almost uncontrollably. But I kept at the sessions, going once a week for several months.

A turning point came when Lynn asked me if I thought my husband would be happier if I lost weight. This was a dangerous question. I really didn't want to go there with him. My biggest fear was not that he'd say "yes," but that he'd say "yes" and I couldn't lose weight. And what if he said "no"? Then what?

I choked up. I didn't know what to say. All indications were that he loved me the way I was, but I was determined to do the work.

That night, with tears streaming down my face, I asked him, "Would you be happier if I lost weight?" Poor guy.

Without hesitation, he replied, "I think *you'd* be happier if you lost weight, and if you were happier, then I'd be happier."

BIG light bulb moment! I didn't want to admit that I'd be happier if I lost weight because that would make my mother right. In my family, fat is bad. Fat people are unhappy, lazy, stupid, ugly, insert the negative adjective of your choice here.

I don't remember exactly when I became overweight, but I remember the first time I felt that there must be something wrong with my body. I was about eight or nine years old and had been to a pediatrician visit with my mother. When we got home, she said to my stepfather, "The doctor said she's chunky." I heard amusement, fear, and disgust all at the same time.

At twelve, I began dieting. Photos of myself from that time don't indicate that I was overweight. Yet, when I read the diary I kept during my high school years, it's filled with pages where I write about feeling like a pig, about hating myself because I ate too much. Then, when I went to college, I really packed on the pounds.

And my mother would say, "You must be unhappy."

So I spent all these years unconsciously trying to prove her wrong. I don't blame my mother; this is just how I rebelled. I could be fat AND happy. I could also be smart, successful, active and lovable. And I was. But then I realized what I was doing – staying fat to prove her wrong – and I thought *how silly is that?*

Of course I knew the health risks associated with being overweight. My mother often told me she was concerned about my health and so that became another thing I had to prove – that I could be overweight AND healthy. For the most part, I was. Yes, my cholesterol was high, but under control with medication; and yes, I had my gall bladder removed; and yes, my back ached, but I rationalized that those things also happen to "skinny" people.

Another thing I quickly realized, along with the need to prove my mother wrong, was that I didn't trust myself. I didn't have much self-confidence and was always looking for approval and validation from others. And even when I got it, it didn't help much. I was an insecure, defensive woman who felt she just wasn't good enough. And that was exactly how I treated myself.

All of these realizations occurred through EFT, and over the course of 18 months, I lost 55 pounds. Along with the weight loss came the confidence to pursue a freelance writing career. In October 2006, I wrote an essay called "Why Weight," which was published in a local women's magazine.

In that essay, I wrote:

I began this quest nearly two years ago. Since then I have lost 55 pounds and have moved from the "obese" category on the Body Mass Index (BMI) chart to the "overweight" category. My goal is to have a "healthy" BMI and that means losing another 20 pounds. I count calories, weigh and measure my food, and exercise, gladly. I can wear "normal sized" clothes and cute shoes. Getting dressed in the morning is a stress-free activity. My body moves more easily and I enjoy challenging myself physically. I have taken up running and participated in a 5K race in May. I enjoy kayaking and hiking, and even household chores are easier.

And my already great marriage is even better. Not because my body is different, but because I am a happier, more confident partner. In fact, I have noticed that my husband is more affectionate with me. I recently told him that I noticed. He agreed but reassured me that it doesn't mean that he didn't love me before, but that I am now more receptive to being loved. He's not more affectionate with me because I am thinner; he's more affectionate with me because I am more affectionate with myself.

I don't lose weight as fast now as I did a year ago and that's okay. Sometimes I need a break from counting calories, sometimes I hit a plateau and sometimes I struggle with that inner rebel. But I don't gain weight. I know that I will reach my goal and maintain my loss forever. And that's because I have made a lifestyle change and because I have done it slowly. Each baby step along the way has become a habit. I have no desire to eat the way I used to, and at the same time I never feel deprived. I am glad there isn't a magic pill or effortless solution because I have learned so much! The process, the experience, and the knowledge I have gained are almost more valuable to me that the pounds I have lost. And yes, I AM happier. (Reprinted with permission from The Day Publishing Company)

I bet you can guess what's coming.

Fast-forward to mid-2008 and I regained 23 of the 55 pounds. Obviously it didn't happen overnight. For a while I maintained my weight loss, give or take five pounds. Then, it was give or take ten pounds. Then my clothes didn't fit, and so on.

How the heck did this happen? I had done it the right way. I had lost weight slowly, I hadn't relied on a fad diet, and I had done the work, damn it! I thought I had it all figured out. I thought I had resolved all my issues around weight. I continued to exercise and my eating habits were certainly not as bad as they used to be…or were they? I had stopped logging my food and exercise, so how could I know for sure? Was I being honest with myself? I wasn't perfect but I also didn't expect myself to be...or did I?

Along with the pounds came panic, shame, frustration, and anger. I wallowed in self-pity a bit, I punished myself a lot, and I was desperate, searching for the magic pill I once never thought I'd want.

Had I stopped caring about myself? Had I stopped nurturing myself? In hindsight, I can now see that I had definitely stopped accepting myself. I think the shift occurred when I went from being happy about having lost 55 pounds to being disappointed that I hadn't lost 76 pounds, which was my original goal. I lost sight of what I had accomplished, and focused only on what I hadn't.

So, as 2008 came to a close, I was in a pretty bad place. Deep down inside I knew that more than anything, more than a diet or a magic pill, what I needed was to love and accept myself.

What I see, in hindsight, is a woman who identified herself as her weight. "I've lost 55 pounds!" That's who I was. I was a "weight loss success story," complete with before and after photos. I was invited to New York City for a professional photo shoot and interview and ended up on the cover of *Quick & Simple*, a weekly women's magazine published by *Good Housekeeping*. Then came a commercial that aired nationally. Those were heady times.

Don't get me wrong. I loved it when someone asked, "How did you do it?" and I'd confidently respond, "Eating right and exercise." I'd watch for the inevitable disappointed reaction – the reaction that said they'd hoped I'd discovered some new and easy solution for weight loss. Then, I'd explain that I'd also done a lot of headwork...you know, the emotional component. I'd explain EFT and how I'd had some "ah-ha" moments, let go of some negative energy, and got down to the business of losing weight.

I also loved the reaction I got from people who knew me "before" – especially because it wasn't just a physical transformation. I felt like my whole being had been transformed. My best friend from childhood, who lives in Arizona and doesn't see me often, put it this way: "My Karen is back. I didn't realize that you'd been gone...that you were hiding yourself." She told me I had a sparkle in my eyes, a spring in my step, and an aura of confidence she hadn't seen in a very long while.

But...

And isn't there always a "but?"...

I never reached my goal.

Yes, I had lost more than 50 pounds, but my original goal was to lose 76 pounds. I was still overweight, according to the BMI chart, and so, deep down inside, I didn't feel worthy of all the attention.

I was also intently comparing myself to my "dieting" friends. Some of them had lost more than I had, some had reached their goal weights, some were going even further and sculpting their bodies, running marathons, and becoming body builders! At the same time, I felt cocky...I had figured it all out and, as I wrote in my essay, "...I don't gain weight. I know that I will reach my goal and maintain my loss forever."

Did that work against me? Do I have more work to do? Am I just fated to be fat? Am I lazy? Do I just not want it bad enough? What's wrong with me?

The thought of re-losing weight feels like a much greater burden than the original 55 pounds. And at the very same time, I know that I can't and *don't* want to view this as a struggle – as a fight to be fought, a battle to be won – because if I do, that's exactly what I'll get. A fight. A battle. A struggle.

In the time since I reached that new low on the scale, I have become aware that I am on a quest for the sweet spot – that balance between healthy body weight and image, and self-acceptance *right now*. But it feels like the harder I look for it, the harder it becomes to find. It's elusive. Kind of like love.

Actually, it's not "kind of like love." It IS love.

Then I came across this quote from author and mythologist Joseph Campbell and I knew it was time to do some more work:

> *"It is by going down into the abyss that we*
> *recover the treasures of life.*
> *Where you stumble, there lies your treasure."*

The first step was signing up for a twelve-week class – "Living Lighter: a Holistic Approach to Weigh Loss" – offered by Amy Martin, a local registered nurse and holistic counselor. The class was described as a way to "get motivated and find inspiration to keep you on track; leave with tools to help you through your week, including menus, logs, and reminders; learn how to keep your metabolism on all day; let go of the emotional blocks that stand in your way; learn self-hypnosis techniques to get your subconscious mind in line with, and supportive of, what you really want; and get started on some physical movement, including isotonic exercises, tai chi, hula-hooping, and more."

My first reaction was, "But I know all of this already! I know how to count calories. I know what healthy food is. I don't need menus, and I exercise at least five times a week."

My second reaction was, "Yeah, I know all of that, but I don't want to do it."

But the idea of being able to let go of emotional blocks and getting my subconscious mind in line with what I really want attracted me. And finally, I realized that taking the class would be my "abyss" – it would be a place to stumble and recover my treasure.

What came out of that class is the basis for this book. It got me started on the next leg of what I now know to be my never-ending journey.

Part I: Living Lighter
January 2009

"Life is but a mass of habits –
practical, emotional, intellectual, systematically organized for our
greatness or our grief."
~ William James

Awareness

I went to the first Living Lighter class with an open mind, even though I was nervous and scared. The Living Lighter scale and my home scale had me at the same weight, so that's a good thing.

Then came the moment I dreaded – setting a goal. That's when the tears started. Setting goals paralyzes me. The minute I set a goal, I feel resistant, powerless and scared. Is it because I feel it is impossible to achieve any goal I set for myself? Or is it because I don't really want this? I got through it, and decided that by the end of the twelve weeks, I would lose at least six pounds.

Class started with a quote by William James: *"Life is but a mass of habits – practical, emotional, intellectual, systematically organized for our greatness or our grief."*

We were told that Week One would be all about awareness and consciousness, "so notice your habits and make notes." Amy then explained the typical thought/response pattern: we have a thought that leads to a feeling, and then our bodies respond.

She asked, "What is the most negative thought you have about this process (letting go of weight)?"

My response: *I'm afraid.*

She asked, "And what feeling comes with that thought?"

My response: *Being afraid makes me feel stupid, lazy, irresponsible, and worthless.*

She continued, "And how does your body feel when you feel that?"

My response: *I feel tense and tight.*

This is awareness. In my notebook I wrote, *what do I think that makes me feel that makes me eat?*

I explored that worthless feeling some more. I view "worthless" as one of several selves. The Worthless Karen wants to hide in her office and not put herself out there because she's afraid of being criticized and judged. And so, the worthless feeling continues.

Amy then suggested turning that feeling around. In response, I wrote, *the fact is, I am brave and valuable AND I am FREE to feel my power and my value!*

Okay, so I wrote it and I could see it, but I am not sure I believed it. I get that I *should* believe it. I *wanted* to believe it.

Meeting My Evil Twins

Awareness happens on many levels and in many forms. Sometimes I think I'm doing everything right, but unless I actively keep track or am reminded to do something, I'm never really sure.

So, thanks to my computer announcing the time each hour, I remember to fill up my glass and I'm drinking more water. I've also begun keeping a food diary again. I know it's a proven, key component of a healthy weight loss plan, but until Living Lighter, I hadn't been willing to do it. Writing down what I eat, along with eating six smaller meals every three to four hours, soothes me. It helps me feel in control. And the deep breathing technique we've learned, along with simple stretches each hour, keeps me calm and grounded. I don't feel so restless.

I'm grateful for these realizations. They help me catch myself sooner. I understand that there will be mistakes and I will have setbacks along the way.

Also, in the name of awareness, I thought I'd get to know some of my different selves, my Evil Twins. We've already met Worthless Karen. There's also Scared Karen, Pissed-Off Karen, Resistant Karen, You-Can't-Make-Me Karen, Reluctant Karen…you get the idea.

What makes Evil Twins so evil is that they hold us back and serve us at the same time. So while Worthless Karen protects me from criticism and judgment, she also holds me back from wanting to set a goal. You-Can't-Make-Me Karen allows me to stay in a comfortable place, but doesn't let me stretch and grow either.

Amy specializes in RoHun Therapy, which includes imagery exercises. You visualize embracing your Evil Twins, telling them they are okay, and letting them go while telling them you don't need them anymore.

I'm looking forward to letting my Evil Twins go, but I'm not ready. I've invested too much time and effort with them. And they seem pretty invested in me as well.

About 4:30 in the afternoon, on a day after the first Living Lighter class, I began to feel restless...wanting to eat something and feeling slightly annoyed and guilty about it. I wanted a glass of wine but there wasn't any in the house. Tim (my husband) won't be home for dinner because he's going to a meeting. Maybe the orange I had for a snack wasn't enough. Should I track my calories?

I don't want to.

Hello, Evil Twin.

When Tim is away, or won't be home at the regular time, I tend to get restless and feel that time is standing still. I hate the endless *blah-blah-blah* in my head. So I sit, feeling paralyzed. I don't want to get up and do anything. I just keep cycling through my email, Facebook, and the message boards I post on. I could get up and exercise. I could do some cleaning. I could do some writing.

But I don't want to.

Hello, Resistant Karen.

The Tortoise And The Hare

I had a moment of clarity.

I have a tendency to be the hare and not the tortoise. It might serve me better to learn to do a little bit each day rather than going all out, becoming too tired or burned out. And that extends into many areas: how fast I eat, how hard I exercise, how quickly I work.

It also reminds me of something my dentist once told me. I had been complaining that my gums were sore, and he said I probably brushed my teeth too hard. Bingo! I used to think that the harder I brushed, the cleaner my teeth would be.

I can be gentle with myself and still have clean teeth.

Slow and steady *can* win the race.

7% (Or Losing Weight In Public)

Oprah once featured guests who were "weight loss success stories" but who had fallen off the wagon, so to speak. The man on the show had lost 214 pounds on *The Biggest Loser* (a show I have never seen), and the woman had lost 50 pounds and become a body builder. The man had regained more than 100 pounds. The woman had also regained some of her weight, and said she had not been to the gym in a very long time.

On the one hand, it's nice to know I'm not alone. On the other hand, it begs the question, "Why? Why can't we keep the weight off?"

I remember reading somewhere that only 7% of the people who lose weight keep it off.

Now, *The Biggest Loser* guy lost a huge amount of weight in a very short time – more than 200 pounds in just eight months! There are plenty of articles out there that describe the pitfalls and hazards of rapid weight loss, from its impact on your health to difficulty maintaining the loss.

I guess that's what makes my slide upsetting to me. I didn't lose it too fast. I didn't take diet pills. I didn't follow a fad diet. I worked on the emotional stuff. I thought I had it all figured out. Maybe that's where I failed. I don't consider myself to be a know-it-all but perhaps, in this case, I *did* think I knew it all.

There's also something about having your weight loss success become a public event, which happened to me. Or rather, if I am honest, I allowed to happen. I'm not blaming being a "weight loss success story" for my regain, but there was a sense of finality...that I reached the pinnacle...that I was done, even though I knew it wasn't true. Maintaining goes on long after the magazine is archived and the applause fades.

I think it must have something to do with the normal highs and lows in life. The higher the high, the greater potential there is for a lower low. And so it all comes back to a more balanced approach. Not just for weight loss, but for having lost the weight and maintaining the loss.

Awareness Has Left The Building

Sometime over the weekend at the end of the first week, I stopped stretching and doing breathing exercises every hour on the hour. But I was aware of this, so I guess that counts for something.

For the weigh-in, I had no expectations. It hadn't been a "perfect" week, but the week wasn't about being perfect. It was about being aware.

And what I became aware of was:

- I like to eat in front of the computer. I know I shouldn't, but I am not willing to make the change at this point.
- I tend to eat too fast.
- If I wait too long, I tend to not exercise.
- As the week went on, I became less excited than I was after the first session.

Psychological Uneasiness

That's what Week Two brought.

How willing am I to put up with the discomfort of depriving myself? The question isn't, "How willing am I to be hungry?" or even "How willing am I to put up with not eating my favorite foods?" It's about being willing to put up with a "bad" feeling and not stuffing my face over it.

It's about "should" versus "could" and "can't" versus "won't."

Unwillingness is often perceived as inability. I CAN deal with the discomfort, but am I WILLING? The truth is I am perfectly able and capable, and if I say, "I can't," I set myself up for failure. There is no power in "I can't." It blinds me to responsibility. "Won't" puts the power – and the responsibility – right back in my hands.

For example, I might say, "I should go to the gym, but I can't," (for whatever reason). That sentence is full of guilt and lacks power. So instead I say, "I could go to the gym, but I won't." Now it's about a choice that I made and responsibility that I took.

So, how do I deal with psychological uneasiness? Awareness!

As part of an exercise, Amy asked us how excess weight serves us.

My response: *Weight protects me from the rejection I might experience if I step into the light.*

Is that my psychological uneasiness? Stepping into the light?

My "homework" was about identifying my psychological discomfort, examining it, and focusing on it; about putting into words what I want; about rating my hunger and the satisfaction I feel when I eat; about being aware of what I'm really hungry for in the big picture; and being aware of what my goal is, weight-wise.

And that led to a bout of psychological irritation.

Part of it had to do with the fact that my scale showed a three-pound loss, but Amy's scale showed only a quarter pound loss. But more than that, I felt impatient during class and not as open to listening as the previous week. I wanted more coaching on my food choices, yet when Amy gave us breakfast smoothie recipes, I thought, *I already know all of this. I get the whole protein thing. I don't need to be told again!*

In addition to being irritated, I was hungry when I got home. Great. I ate something that should have satisfied me, but it didn't. What I really want to do was stuff my face.

While digging through the layers of uneasiness and irritation, I remembered that one of the things I am "hungry" for is to be heard…to be recognized. I got some of that during class, but I wanted more. Sometimes I feel like a little kid saying, "Look at me, look at me! Watch me!"

So, it was two kinds of hunger: I was truly hungry because I hadn't eaten since 7:30 that morning, but the desire to stuff my face was about something else. I recognized a bit of psychological uneasiness. When I feel hungry, I often have a guilty or angry reaction, like I shouldn't be hungry. I don't like to be hungry. Being hungry makes me think I am weak. But maybe that's because I don't trust myself to eat only what I need.

Cut Soda, Add Whole Grains

Duh!

You can't open a magazine or click on a web site without reading an article about how to "shed those extra pounds," and they all have advice like "stop drinking soda and add whole grains."

And I'm thinking, "But I don't drink soda, and I already eat whole grains!"

Then I thought about all those little bad habits that have crept back in. Like when eating out, having fries or chips, or partaking of the bread that's brought to the table before the meal.

I knew I wouldn't miss those things, so that became a concrete step I felt comfortable taking.

The Trickster And My Core Of Rot

Remember the thought/feeling/reaction exercise from Week One?

It's time to put it into practice, because The Trickster is trying to make a deal with me that might make me feel better in the short term, but not the long term.

The Trickster is that aspect of ourselves that will help us out of a sticky or uncomfortable situation…but always at a price.

What's my faulty thought? "I am a show off. I am selfish. I am a spoiled brat. Just who do I think I am?"

How do I feel as a result? "I feel anger, annoyance, guilt, impatience, disappointment, and frustration."

How does this hurt me? "It makes me hide. It makes me pull back."

How does persisting in this thought serve me? "It protects me from criticism and rejection."

The Trickster senses my weakness, and slides out of the shadows. I make a deal with him.

"I can't deal with rejection and criticism. Can you help me?"

The Trickster says, "Of course! I'll keep you safe from rejection and criticism, but in return you'll be frustrated and sad, and you will overeat to temporarily feel better."

Is this the deal I want? No!

Turning around my negative thoughts, I tell myself, "I am free to feel the beauty, the light, and the strength within me, and I am free to express it. I have everything I need inside."

If only it were as easy to do it as it is to say it. That's where my Core of Rot is.

The Core of Rot is an idea developed by Charles Seashore. It's that part of ourselves that disgusts us, whether deservedly or not. And the Core of Rot will keep growing if we keep adding to it.

Remember when I spoke about feeling irritated after last week's class? And why? After admitting my irritation, I felt as if I'd been a bad girl for wanting attention and even for having been irritated. It's childhood crap, and that's what makes it so insidious.

The women in my family were raised to be seen and not heard. Their natural abilities were not valued, and sometimes even squelched. "Don't rock the boat," they were told. "Don't be a show-off."

Somewhere along the line I made a decision about myself – a decision that I am a spoiled brat. And because of that decision, I hide myself so as not to get too much attention, to not shine too brightly because then I'd not only be a spoiled brat, I'd be a spoiled brat that was showing off. I hide by using food...and I'm fat because everyone knows it's impossible for fat people to shine, right?

So I felt irritated for feeling like I needed attention during the class, and that led to a whole cascade of negative thoughts that the Trickster was more than happy to help me deal with...for a price, of course. I don't feel selfish and spoiled all the time, and it's not something I feel about myself regularly, but there are moments when I believe I'm behaving like a spoiled child. The negative messages all pile up and become part of our ever-growing Core of Rot.

But I was able to turn it around...to put into practice the thought/feeling/response lesson and illustrate for myself that it can be done.

I Am An Onion

I had a good cry watching Oprah one afternoon. Several overweight/obese children and teens, and their parents, were taking part in an "intervention." Part of the show involved having the kids say to their parents, "I am angry that..." Fill in the blank. One of the therapists facilitating the interventions said that it's really important for parents to give their children a safe space in which to be angry...even when they're angry with their parents. And their parents were told to not be defensive or critical.

One of the girls said to her mom, "I am so angry that you think this is your fault." "This" being her body, her weight, which she pointed at as she said it.

I'll never forget when my mother said it was "such a relief" for her to realize that I may "just be addicted to carbs." This was in the 90s, when low-carb diets became popular. She said something like, "I'm just glad it's not my fault." I also remember hearing her talk to my grandmother about my weight when I was a child, and saying, "It's not my fault." I felt like I was a mistake.

A lot of kids on the show said things like, "I am angry that Dad left us" and "I am angry that my mother is sick and can't take care of us." And even though it occurred more than 40 years ago - when I was just two years old - I recognize that my parents' divorce still saddens me deeply. And then it pisses me off that it STILL BOTHERS ME! I thought I had it all figured out. I thought I had worked it out. I thought I understood it.

How freaking long will it be an issue?!

I never felt safe being angry or upset when I was a kid because I never knew what reaction I'd get from the adults. In fact, there were times when I didn't want to hurt my parents' feelings by bringing up my anger or sadness. Sometimes the response would be a dismissive "I'm sorry you feel that way" or "I tried to do the best I could."

My perception of the past is just that – my perception. And that's not saying that I felt unsafe much of the time or unloved, because that's not true. I realize now that the safest place I have is within myself, but not if I'm being angry with myself for having these "negative" feelings.

And that leads to what Week Four was all about: eating intuitively and looking at what gets in the way of trusting myself to do so. This is BIG. Because I DON'T trust myself. Week Four was also about forgiving myself for needing to re-resolve what I consider to be really old stuff.

Making A Bad Choice On Purpose

Have you ever made a bad choice on purpose? I'm not talking being confronted with two choices and choosing the one you probably shouldn't just to see what would happen. I'm talking about knowing you're making a bad choice and doing it anyway.

Tim was away on business for a day or two, and I consciously made bad choices about food (can we say "carb fest?") and ate too much. I actually planned it all out ahead of time and went shopping for the express purpose of bingeing. And as I made these choices I realized I felt like I was getting away with something.

Why do I feel the need to binge when Tim is away for a day or two? And what's the difference between eating in response to stress/anger/sadness and what I call "happy eating" – eating in response to feeling good?

At least I'm *aware*, right??

Do You Have Sex Every Time You Think About It?

Mark Bittman, the *New York Times* columnist and author of *Food Matters: A Guide to Conscious Eating*, was a guest of Tom Ashbrook on NPR. During the interview, Bittman made an interesting comment about "being with hunger":

"You don't have sex every time you think about it; you don't take a nap every time you feel a little tired, so why grab something to eat every time you feel a little hungry?"

He went on to talk about people needing to eat in the afternoon before dinner and how, for many, grabbing something to eat means having a candy bar, a slice of pizza, or both, versus, say, having an apple, a handful of nuts, or some popcorn.

I'd like to say that I fall in to the latter group, but often, what actually happens is that I virtuously eat the apple or nuts, then follow it up with something much less virtuous. But in the bigger picture, what I see is a society that has to have food available at every turn. God forbid we get a little hungry.

Spotlight On Karen

I was the only one in class at the beginning of Week Five so I got all the attention. I was relishing the fact that I'd be able to go deeper into myself with no distractions. As painful as this work can sometimes be, I don't shy away from it. So bring it on!

Amy and I talked about my week and specifically the fact that I tend to binge when Tim goes out of town. I observed that Tim seems to provide the structure to my life, and that without him I can't take care of myself, that I can't function (not literally, this is just the basic feeling I had).

Amy asked, "So, does Tim equal structure? What does your structure look like?"

The negative side of structure, to me, is that it's limiting. Boring. No freedom and no flow. There's rebellion associated with it – or the need for rebellion.

The positive side of structure, to me, is that it provides safety, guidelines, and schedules. A compass. An evaluation tool.

I am not against structure. I appreciate the role it plays in my life. But why does Tim represent structure to me?

As we talked, Amy asked me about the "structure" I have built for myself. It has walls made of judgment, weight problems, money problems, fear, addictive behaviors, guilt, and a critical voice. I see myself as the prisoner within those walls. My belief

– my faulty belief – is that the walls of my structure help me control myself. I believe the only way to have self-control is to have those walls around me – they keep me from getting out, and other elements from getting in.

So is there another type of structure that might foster self-acceptance and self-control? A structure without the whips and chains?

I started to see that it's irrational to try and get what I want surrounded by my current structure. I needed to build a new one, because the current one isn't serving me anymore.

At one time, it did serve me, because it kept me from going overboard with shopping, drugs, alcohol, and even eating to a certain extent. Even though I have dabbled in addiction, so to speak, I've never let it go too far. The old structure served me, but it didn't help me love and accept myself. I kept myself inside so I wouldn't go overboard, and in exchange, I paid the price with my lack of: self-confidence, inner peace, health, self-expression, and self-acceptance.

What might my new structure look like? Self-acceptance is at its center. The walls are made of forgiveness, love, honor for myself and my feelings, gentleness with myself, and peace.

So when Tim goes away, I will still make choices, but what voice will I use? What will the origin of those choices be? My voice can be critical and judgmental, or it can be loving and gentle. It can come from a place of imprisonment or freedom. All of this fits in with what I've been revealing to myself already – but it does add reinforcement. And it lays the cornerstone for a new structure.

Up. Down. Up. Down...Up.

I was nervous going into class at the start of Week Six. The scale was up at home. Sure enough, Amy's scale showed I'd gained as well - 2.75 pounds. Sadness, frustration, and a sense that nothing will work and "I can't do this" overwhelmed me. I couldn't stop crying...crying like a distraught little girl.

Then, I was off to my annual physical. I held it together as I refused to be weighed by the assistant. When my doctor came in, I couldn't hold it back, and I cried some more. She was great, though, and supportive of Living Lighter.

Afterward, I went grocery shopping, feeling fragile and drained. Crushed, even. The number on the scale has so much power over me. When I got home, I cried some more.

I was hungry, but felt chastised. Like a good girl, I ate a tangerine. I didn't feel like bingeing. In fact, I felt the opposite. I made some tea and noted that the kitchen was a mess. And I still hadn't unpacked the groceries. I had that "I'm a bad girl" feeling, and it compelled me to clean the kitchen. As I thought about it, an old feeling or fragment of memory came to the surface: I should be punished, either by myself or someone else. I felt like I should be ashamed and send myself to my room, as if I am still a little girl.

Part of it is this: Tim isn't home, so I don't have to clean up after myself. I can do it when I want to. When Tim is home, I clean up. If I don't, he'll automatically clean up after me. I hate it. It makes me feel like I have to do it so he won't. He has enough to do. He never complains or says anything negative; it's just who he is. He just does it naturally.

And then I feel guilty. It's almost like I'd rather he complain!

It's almost like I can't take care of myself unless someone is nagging me to do it!

Is that where my motivation comes from? From shame and guilt? Was I brought up that way?

When I was a kid, there was always a sense of freedom and "I can do whatever I want" when my parents weren't home. Let the dishes pile up. Eat what and when I want. Was I so tightly controlled that this was the inevitable outcome? Or am I just a lazy, selfish adult child?

When I supposedly grew up and lived on my own, that was how I lived! I mean, I certainly did clean up after myself, and my apartments weren't dirty or even that messy. But there was no one telling me what to do or when to do it, and I liked it. Sometimes I didn't do the dishes right away. I especially hated washing utensils, since I didn't have a dishwasher, and sometimes I'd let them sit for too long. Ick.

It wasn't responsible of me to be that way, but who cared? It was just me.

This comes back to that whole conversation with Amy about structure, and what does my structure look like? And how it's not so easy to shed the old and don the new, even when you're aware!

So, I felt that cycle of shame, and the shame motivating me to do the right thing, which, in this case, was cleaning up the kitchen. Then I felt a bit self-righteous. Then I felt a lot better. And with that feeling came the desire to eat – to dig in with delight and glee and distraction.

I know for a lot of people stress, anger, and sadness can make them turn to food. For me, it comes afterward…when I start to feel better, when the feelings of guilt and shame subside.

Riding The Tiger

After a final intense cry, I got a good night's sleep and felt stronger and more sure of myself the next day. Even though I'd been so distraught during the previous class, I picked up some useful tools.

The focus of the class had been about reminding ourselves of where we want to go and how we want to get there. Some trips are relatively easy (for example, to the store) and others are a little more daunting (for example, driving from Connecticut, where I am, to California).

When you are intent on getting where you're going, especially on a long trip, you have to say "no" to distractions along the way – even if they seem like a good idea at the time. You have to decide what's more important – getting to California or stopping in Vegas for a couple of days.

So, where am I going?

When Amy asked my destination, I said, "I want to get back to Wow," recalling the feeling I got when I ran for the first time.

It was September of 2005 and I was taking a walk to the beach. A thought bubbled up. *I can run if I want to.* Before I could think about it further, my body responded to the signal sent by my brain, and I ran. I didn't run fast or far, but I ran!

I will never forget what went through my mind in that moment: *No matter what happens, I will be okay. I can take care of myself.*

I finally had a clear understanding of how strong I really am, and I had a stunning realization: *Now I know what it feels like to love and accept myself.*

That's what Wow felt like the first time around. So maybe saying that I want to "get back to Wow" implies a step backwards. So I'll rephrase it and say, "I'm on a journey to the New Wow, but I haven't forgotten what that first Wow felt like." I think it's important to remind myself that I know what Wow feels like despite indications to the contrary.

On the most elemental level, my goal is to feel wonderful about myself, because from there, all power and goodness flows. So each and every day (sometimes every hour) I have to ask myself if what I am doing is taking me closer to "wow" or if it is a detour.

One of the tools Amy gave us is a tai chi sequence called "Embrace the Tiger, Return to Mountain." The Tiger represents a challenge and the Mountain represents home (heart). The sequence involves looking at everything around you with "the soft eyes of acceptance."

In other forms of martial arts, "riding the tiger" means having courage. It's interesting that in tai chi, the Tiger represents a challenge. Maybe, in this light, to "Embrace the Tiger" is accepting the challenge and letting it take you where it wants to go. When I think about what my "Tiger" is, I realize it's myself. I am my challenge.

What a coincidence that my Chinese horoscope sign is the Tiger!

We also did another exercise in that class that involved naming the emotions around self-sabotage, naming the faulty thoughts behind these emotions, and naming how they serve us or hinder us. As I blurted out my answers, I realized they were all pretty much the same answers from other similar exercises.

The emotions: self-doubt, self-criticism, fear, judgment.

The faulty thoughts: I can't do this; it will never work.

How they serve me: if I don't do it, I can just stay safe and do what I want

Why is safety important? Because it keeps me from failing, or from being criticized for failing. And believe me, as I see it in writing, I'm aware of the paradox!

What other ways can I feel safe? How can I reward myself and keep my focus on getting to Wow?

I think what I felt was old guilt that surfaces under superficial circumstances. It's like an iceberg: there's a small part that sticks up above the surface, and there's a gigantic part under the surface. There are times when I honestly feel that I am okay just the way I am, and other times when I feel that I am deeply flawed and a bad person. I haven't yet figured out what triggers one feeling versus the other.

I can see my cycles. I don't think I could sustain this type of deep introspection over too long a period, but I have done it a few times. I'm not sure how long is too long, but when I look back, I realize that this is just how I do it. I have periods of intense introspection and periods of processing it, then periods of just "being" with it, and finally I just "am" for a while.

Hypnosis And Hula Hoops

Week One: -0.25 pounds
Week Two: +3.25 pounds
Week Three: -0.75 pounds
Week Four: -1.50 pounds
Week Five: +2.75 pounds
Week Six: -4.00 pounds

Yep, down four pounds! What's interesting is that the class discussion that followed weigh-in was exactly what I'd needed to hear…because my immediate (faulty) thought upon stepping on the scale was, "Well, the scale will be up again. It's inevitable. That's the pattern." But I didn't say it aloud until later.

Amy asked how my week was and, in light of the loss, I said, "Uh, it looks like it was a pretty good week!" I'd made good choices, dealt with my psychological uneasiness, didn't deprive myself, exercised, and felt a lot of peace around food. I'd journaled consistently too, but there was also a sense of not trusting it. The reality is that I was lucky, not that I had worked at it.

This Week Six class presented self-hypnosis as a tool for getting the unconscious mind to align with conscious desires.

Amy asked me to write down what my conscious mind wants – such as "living lighter" – and what my unconscious mind is telling me – such as "I can't do this," "I don't want to change," or "I don't want to try."

I wrote: *I am down four pounds this week but I'll be up again next week* and *I want to live lighter, but I don't want to try. I want to take the easy way out.*

We talked about traditional cognitive therapy, which has, as its premise:

"...our thoughts, even though we may be unaware of them, precede our emotional responses, and that if we can exercise control over our thoughts, we can change dysfunctional emotional patterns. Cognitive theory says that our automatic thoughts stem from fundamental attitudes that we hold at the edge of conscious awareness, and they, in turn, evolved from core beliefs that have developed from our interchanges with our environment, others and ourselves, from the moment of birth. The most powerful of these beliefs are thought to become entrenched early in life, as deeply embedded patterns of response." (Instant Emotional Healing: Acupressure for the Emotions by Peter Lambrou and George Pratt)

Amy then outlined four steps to self-hypnosis:

1. Relax. (Did you know that the only difference between relaxation and hypnosis is intent?)
2. Begin to visualize yourself in your happiest, healthiest state. What does it look like? Breathe it in, feel it, look into the eyes of that happiest, healthiest self. Use all your senses to "see" that self.
3. Give yourself motivating suggestions about what foods and exercises will be best for your body.
4. Align your unconscious thoughts with your conscious desires.

Amy suggested doing this once a day for ten to twenty minutes. I have to admit that I immediately thought, "But I don't want to do self-hypnosis once a day; I want someone to do it to me! Besides I haven't been doing all those other things you suggested, like breathing and stretching every hour (although I was doing them more than I used to). Now I have to do this too?"

Just slap me now.

So what do I say to align my unconscious thoughts with my conscious desires?

"I am free to see the scale decreasing?"

"The scale just keeps moving down, effortlessly?"

Or how about, "My effort brings me joy" AND "I am committed to aligning my unconscious mind with my conscious desires."

Next, Amy got out some hula-hoops and gave us each one to take home. She said it's a lot of fun, provides a bit of a cardio workout, and is good for core strengthening.

We tried them out and, sure enough, she was right!

This Is What Victory Looks Like

Since the previous class, I'd been both "at peace with food" and somewhat uneasy. I realize that the moment I get comfortable with the idea that I'm doing well, I start wanting to make a deal with myself.

Tim is out of town. The first day was no problem; it was the kind of day I'd like to have every day. I woke up naturally at 7 a.m. Had breakfast and coffee while I caught up on email and the news. Went for a brisk forty-minute walk. Came home and showered. Got some work done. Went to a networking luncheon where I made good food choices without effort, and enjoyed connecting with other women. Returned to my office and worked some more. I ate dinner when I was hungry. I played on Facebook for a bit, watched television, read, then went to bed and slept for eight-plus hours.

Day two started out pretty much the same way. I took two back-to-back kickboxing classes for the pure enjoyment of it – not because I felt like I *had* to, and not because I was desperate to burn calories. I notice that my intent makes the difference when I exercise. If I force myself to workout harder because I feel guilty about eating something, I don't have as much fun and I am more likely to hurt myself.

In the afternoon, however, I started thinking about dinner and had the following conversation with myself:

"Hmm...what should I plan for dinner? I'm rather hungry right now. What would be good? Ooo...there's a package of organic, all-natural, whole wheat macaroni and cheese in the cabinet."

"But eating a whole box of macaroni and cheese? Remember the last time I did that? It wasn't all that long ago, and I didn't feel very good – emotionally or physically – afterward."

"Okay. So I need to go to the store, and while I'm out, I'll get some good protein to go with the mac and cheese. But wait...going to the store in this frame of mind might not be a good thing. I'll be tempted. Goldfish crackers...Smartfood popcorn...Smarties..."

"Ooo...Smartfood. A small bag won't hurt."

"Do I really need to go to the grocery store today? What else can I do? What else do I need to do?"

"Well, I have to go to the bank, and I could go to the mall and see what's on sale, even though I don't want to buy any clothes right now because I want to lose some weight. Still, we're going to Florida in a couple of weeks and I'm afraid my warm-weather clothes from last year won't fit."

"I think going to the bank and then the mall is a better idea than going to the store right now."

"Okay."

So I went to the bank, then the mall, and I tried on a bunch of clothes that didn't fit the way I wanted them to. I didn't buy anything because I was pissed off. Clothes just don't fit like they used to and I'm not going to spend money on clothes that don't look and feel great!

Then, on the way home…

"Well, I still don't have a plan for dinner. I want something satisfying and healthy. I really don't want to eat the mac and cheese; it just has too many carbs. Maybe I could stop somewhere and get take-out."

"Oh, there's Ocean Pizza! They make a great grilled chicken salad! Perfect!"

I bought the salad (no dressing), and at home, I put it in a nice bowl, added some fresh cabbage and carrots, and really enjoyed my dinner.

This is what victory looks like.

Inconsistency

During Week Eight, I looked at what might still be standing in my way. How completely do I believe in myself and in my ability to reach my goals?

I think about what I've achieved so far – not in terms of a number on the scale, but in terms of "non-scale" victories, how I feel inside. I want to feel that nothing's standing in my way, and I'm 100% able to accomplish my goals. But I don't feel that way.

The quick answer is that I am inconsistent.

The deeper issue is that in my core I believe I am a quitter, that I can't finish what I start. And I know that having this belief makes it a self-fulfilling prophecy.

Amy asked me what inconsistency physically feels like. I replied that it feels like a huge weight on my shoulders.

What is the opposite of inconsistency? Consistency, of course. But I have an immediate and visceral reaction to the idea, because in my mind it equals mind-numbing boredom. It's also hard and takes effort and control. Kind of like "structure."

My basic faulty thought is: "I'm inconsistent, so I can't get what I want. Why don't I want something if it takes effort? Why is effort the enemy?" During Week Seven, I'd said "my effort brings me joy" in order to align my unconscious thoughts with my conscious desires. But in the intervening seven days, I self-hypnotized *once*.

There's that inconsistency thing again.

Maybe consistency isn't the opposite of inconsistency. Maybe it's more about clarity versus confusion. I'll be the first to admit that when I'm confused, it usually means I'm avoiding something, which usually results in inconsistent behavior.

So my homework is to write a self-hypnosis script that works for me and to conclude with an affirmation that I believe 100%...that makes me feel I can absolutely accomplish my goal, no doubt about it.

I stalled for a while, partly because I've been afraid I won't be able to do it...that there's nothing I can think or say that will fit those criteria. Eventually I created Karen's Self-Hypnosis Script.

> *"As I breathe in, I breathe in peace and clarity.*
> *As I exhale, I exhale out inconsistency and confusion.*
> *In my happiest, healthiest state, I feel free in my body,*
> *My clothes slip easily onto my body,*
> *I feel strong and tight,*
> *My skin glows and I exude peace and contentment.*
>
> *I eat wonderful, colorful, crunchy vegetables;*
> *Naturally sweet and colorful fruits;*
> *Yummy lean protein and healthful whole grains and nuts.*
>
> *I am clear about who I am and what I want and my commitment to myself.*
> *My effort brings me joy."*

Why I Refuse To Eat Foods I Don't Like

Amy asked if we ever eat foods we don't like. One of the other women in the class said her husband likes Brussels sprouts, and since he does all the cooking, she will eat them even though she doesn't particularly care for them.

My immediate reaction was an incredulous, "Why would you eat something you don't like??"

Then some not-so-nice memories surfaced. When I was a child, I was forced to eat foods I didn't like. Lima beans. Liver. Mashed potatoes. Peas. It was a texture thing. Those foods made me gag. And it wasn't about "just trying" the food, it was about eating all of it, even though I'd tried these foods before and truly did not like them. Sometimes I'd gag, spit it back up, and be forced to eat that. Or I was threatened with having to eat it for breakfast the next morning. I was told I was spoiled, that there were starving children in the world.

You-Can't-Make-Me Karen was born around this time. Of course, I wouldn't have dared say "you can't make me" to them. But You-Can't-Make-Me Karen got back at them by sneaking or stealing the foods she liked and eating too much of them.

I think I let her go somewhere around the middle of the Living Lighter program. All along I've been meeting these different versions of myself – the Evil Twins who have served me in some ways but who have also held me back. I look forward to meeting them, and then saying goodbye.

Wow Has Left The Building

I got on the scale at home for the first time in about two weeks and hadn't gained or lost, and I was okay with that. I got on the scale the next day and was UP three pounds. I thought, "I just can't deal with getting on Amy's scale today. I just can't."

I started down that familiar path of self-pity: this will never work. But my heart wasn't really into the trip. Instead, I looked more objectively at the past two weeks – what I'd done right (consistently) as well as the choices that might not have been the best.

Here's what I did consistently...or at least, what worked for me.

- Choosing fresh veggies and fruit for snacks.
- Eating more slowly, to the point that I'm finishing after Tim, and as a result...
- Eating less at dinner
- Exercising

Choices that might not have been the best (or, what didn't work form me):

- Carbohydrates
- Wine
- Carbs
- Carbs with too much sodium

I arrived at the Living Lighter class feeling a little defensive, but in control and wanting to be honest and objective. When I said I didn't want to get on the scale, Amy was fine with it. She said, "This is about the wisdom of everything you know combined with the immense self-love and self-care." And I think anyone who is on this journey – the journey of self-acceptance – understands that it's not about what you know or don't know. It's about self-love.

As part of the class, Amy asked us to do a "Negative Emotion Dump." She wanted us to write out all of our frustrations, upsets, anger, sadness, and so on. After five minutes of dumping, we shredded our thoughts. Literally. She got out a paper shredder and in they went. Whiiirrrrr. And they were gone.

Why Putting On A Happy Face Isn't Always the Best Thing To Do

Affirmations.

Smile though your heart is breaking.

Think positive!

Turn that frown upside down!

We all get it. A positive attitude attracts positive events. But I also believe there's nothing gained from denying what we consider to be negative emotions.

In fact, I read a book called *ElderWoman: Reap The Wisdom, Feel The Power, Embrace the Joy* by Marian Van Eyk McCain that mentioned the phenomenon of "radical aliveness." It means remaining fully open to all experiences, whether pleasant or painful. The idea isn't new. The concept has been around for thousands of years – "radical aliveness" is just a new way to express it.

When you're radically alive, you embrace everything within your experience, rather than judging experiences as either "bad" or "good." You willingly accept pain and confusion and all the other negative feelings, and acknowledge that they are as meaningful, relevant, and full of learning potential as your joyful ones.

So when Amy brought up the idea that "trying to be positive" is not always the best solution, I was interested. She went so far as to say that denying negative emotions is a form of self-abuse. It's silly to put a smile on your face when what you really need to do is acknowledge feelings you might view as ugly.

I get that. It's not only okay for me to reveal my shadow side, it's actually an act of love to do so! And this whole deal – this whole process – is about making choices between self-love and self-abuse.

Amy said, "Affirmations can be as ineffective as putting a smiley face on an empty gas tank. You're not going anywhere until you fill up the tank." She led us through another Negative Emotion Dump and visualization exercise.

She asked where in our bodies we felt tension as we wrote down the negatives. I felt it in my throat. She asked us to visualize removing the tension, and cradling it in our arms as if it were a baby. My first thought was that I am not a very good cradler. I don't have kids and I usually feel awkward around them. Nurturing just doesn't come naturally to me. But I went with it, and Amy said to imagine soothing a tired, hungry baby who has a wet diaper.

"I know you're tired, hungry, wet, and uncomfortable, but it's okay to feel that way. You will be okay...there, there...I love you and you will be okay."

Wow. As I sat there with my shadow self in my arms, I realized that I don't have much patience with myself...that I get easily annoyed with me. I also realized that I don't have much patience for others, especially in certain circumstances, like illness.

And I acknowledged that some of the women in my family were not particularly patient or accepting either. My discomfort, my sadness, my anger – any "negative" emotion – tended to overwhelm, upset, or annoy them. I got the impression that they had no patience for it.

So, what *is* self-love? Patience. Acceptance. Kindness. Acknowledgment. Softness.

What is self-abuse? Impatience. Judging. Meanness. Annoyance. Denial. Harshness.

How can you tell if you might be self-abusive? One way is to acknowledge when you're impatient, judgmental, or annoyed with someone else. Oh boy...talk about holding the mirror up to myself.

Getting My Kicks

In June 2008, I started Muay Thai kickboxing classes. I signed up at the local dojo (martial arts school) in an act of desperation, thinking I needed to change up my workout. Prior to that, I'd been doing a lot of running and strength training. Then as I started to gain weight, I started pushing myself harder because – although I didn't see it at the time – I'd gone into desperation mode. And I injured myself. Running became more difficult and I wasn't focused on allowing my injuries to heal. So I signed up for kickboxing, and proceeded to gain another ten pounds.

It's the desperation, stupid. I've come to believe that anything we do out of desperation is destined to backfire – in a spectacular fashion.

It's not that I don't love kickboxing. I do. But for a while, I wasn't doing it for the right reasons. It was just a means to an end – I'd beat those pounds off of me. And the more weight I gained, the more desperate I became, so I returned to old behaviors like binge eating. And the cycle continued.

Having taken several metaphorical deep breaths, I decided to take it easier. I kickbox for the sheer joy of it. Damn it.

Reminder To Self

*As I breathe in, I breathe in patience, consistency,
and clarity.*

*As I exhale, I exhale out impatience, inconsistency,
and confusion.*

*In my happiest, healthiest state, I feel free. My clothes slip easily onto
my body.*

*I feel strong and tight. My skin glows, and I exude peace
and contentment.*

*I eat wonderful, colorful, crunchy vegetables…naturally sweet and
colorful fruits…yummy lean protein…and healthful whole grains
and nuts.*

*I move my body in ways that bring me joy and exhilaration, strength
and vitality.*

*I am clear about who I am, what I want, and my commitment to
myself. My effort brings me joy.*

My Truth In Three Acts

So it's Week Ten and I'm not even close to my six-pound weight loss goal. Remember? I was petrified that first day because I didn't want to set a goal. Past experience shows me that the very act of setting a goal means I won't achieve it. *(Is this the Truth?)*

The class started the same way as all the others, with Amy asking, "how are you?" Up until the moment I arrived, I felt pretty good, even though I hadn't lost any weight. I honestly felt that I'd made good progress, but it just hadn't shown up on the scale yet. And I believed that it *would* show up on the scale – sooner rather than later.

Amy suggested that my body might need to be "surprised" – that my metabolism was assuming I would continue to eat the same general way I always had. So I needed to surprise my body by doing something different. And I knew there were a couple of ways I could do that.

At the same time, I felt weepy, frustrated, and angry. I'd been making better choices. I'd been mindful and in control. I also knew I hadn't been perfect, and I also knew this wasn't about being perfect. And now, with Amy's suggestion, I felt I was going to have to give some things up completely if I was ever going to lose any weight! HOW MUCH FREAKING MORE DO I HAVE TO GIVE UP?!

Amy boiled down what I was feeling into "I must deprive myself." *(Is this the Truth?)*

That's when I remembered the internal dialogue I'd had the previous week. I'd been thinking about foods I believe I have no control over. I thought about whether or not it's TRUE that I have no control. *(Is this the Truth?)*

I imagined buying a bag of Goldfish crackers and putting it in the cupboard. I imagined eating just a few and putting the rest away. For a little while, I thought, "Yes, of course I can do that." It was intriguing to think that I could do that.

And I thought about all the conversations I'd ever had with other women who are on this same journey and how many of us believe we have no control.

It's societal and it's systemic. But it's not true.

This Is My Core Of Rot

The time has come, once again, to let go of my frustrated, angry self. I am more ready than in the past...and I know that I'm going to have to do this over and over and over again.

I'd mentioned earlier examining my Core of Rot...looking at that part I consider to be ugly and icky. My shadow self. I've written about the power of acknowledging it, of rolling back the rug to see what's been swept underneath, and looking at it with love and acceptance.

While visualizing the frustrated, angry self, I decided to acknowledge another self. A self that had been front and center in my mind, but one I did not want to acknowledge. I think I'll call her the Gatekeeper of my Core of Rot.

I saw the self who believes she will fall into the family pattern of drinking to the point of drunkenness every day. I saw the self who is critical of those in her family who drink too much. I saw the self who would drink wine every day if it were in the house (one of those things I can't control?)...the self who drinks wine several times a week.

This is the self driving me crazy because she thinks enjoying wine means she's just like those family members. And if she decides *not* to drink wine for a week, to surprise her body and see if those extra calories make a difference, she is afraid someone will point a finger at her and say, "Then you must have a problem." And it will make her defensive, just like those family members.

This is my Core of Rot. It's the fear that I am my family and will end up just like them, numbing myself with alcohol to the point where I can't talk coherently or remember conversations. It's cracking open a door to something I've been afraid to talk about for fear of being judged. Because I judge them, and they judge each other, and it's all a bunch of finger pointing, criticism, and attacks.

I am not my family.

I Am That Which I Desire

I realized again – for the 1,784,014th time – that I don't have to be thin in order to be happy. I can be happy right now. And that, my friends, is what Week Eleven, and the rest of my life, are all about.

Or, as Amy put it, I am understanding and using neural plasticity to empower my health goals.

You see, we have these things in our brains called dendrites. Wikipedia's definition says, "Dendrites are the branched projections of a neuron that act to conduct the electrochemical stimulation received from other neural cells to the cell body, or soma, of the neuron from which the dendrites project."

Another way to understand dendrites is to see that they are how we get stuck in ruts. The good news is that we can also use them to create new and improved ruts...or perhaps "groove" is a better word. Yeah – it's how you get your groove back!

We all have literal ruts in our brains, that we ourselves created. For example, I have an "I can't do it" rut. I created this rut by having that thought over and over and over again, so much so that my dendrites created a physical path in my brain that makes it easier for the thought to become reality...to become part of my physical body.

So it's true – we are what we think! What we see depends mainly on what we look for. How we feel depends mainly on what we think. And, according to something I read by Dr. Christiane Northrup, recent research in quantum physics shows that our *perceptions* about our environment, *not our genes*, determine the quality of our health.

If you focus on strength, flexibility, and good health, you will attract those qualities into your life and body. Dwelling on illness, fear, disease, and pain do just the opposite. It pays to notice and change your thoughts accordingly.

So how do you form a new connection? Create a new "of-course-I-can-do-it" groove?

One way is to use positive "I am" statements over and over and over so you can erase the old rut and create a new groove.

Another way is to understand the constructs of your life. You can figure out what your constructs are by filling in the blank: "In my life, I have learned by experience that…"

For example, I might say, "In my life, I have learned by experience that I can't lose weight and keep it off."

And over time, as I've proven that construct to myself time and again, the dendrites have created a rut in my brain, and now my entire body believes – on a cellular level – that I can't lose weight and keep it off.

Another example: "In my life, I have learned by experience that if I am fat, I must not be very happy."

But wait a minute! I AM really happy, so this must not be true!

The beauty is in the fact that I can change my mind, just like that.

I am fit!

I am light!

I am happy!

I am terrific!

I am fabulous!

I am healthy!

I am Wow!

I am...that!

I am that which I desire!

Amy made a great point with this question: *why do we use pain as a motivator?* Why do we just plod along until we feel pain, then decide in that moment of duress to do something about it? I mean, I know what it's like to plod along feeling pretty good, then catch a glimpse of my reflection and think, "Ugh! I am fat." And then I am moved to action. Maybe.

What if we use our desire for a lighter, more joyful life as motivation?

Hello, Opened Eyes!

"And the day came when the risk it took to
remain tightly closed in a bud
was more painful that the risk it took to bloom."
~ Anais Nin

I remembered this quote as I ran to the beach and saw a flower blooming – the first one after winter. I remembered what it felt like when I took the risk to bloom, and the pain of remaining a tightly closed bud. Right now it feels like I am half closed bud and half bloom…not sure what I want.

Earlier in the week, I'd committed myself to counting and logging my calories at least six days a week. Eating intuitively and mindfully are wonderful, but I need to rediscover what that really means and to do that, I need to see it on paper. It's also a small way for me to get past my fear of – and resistance to – setting a goal.

Funny…I recently read that in addition to being the Constitution State, Connecticut is also "The Land of Steady Habits." Hmmm.

Then a friend of mine put this oldie-but-a-goody out there:

"The definition of insanity is doing the same thing over and over
again and expecting different results."
~ Albert Einstein

And you know what? I realize that this is exactly what I've been doing: eating the same old, same old, and expecting to lose weight. I had cut back and begun making better choices, but it was only enough to stop me from gaining. It wasn't enough to get lighter! Hello, opened eyes!

That's one of the reasons I love to run: it's moving meditation. It's opened eyes. It's about what I can do, not what I can't. It's being in half bloom and being okay with it. It's crying at the beauty of it all.

Reinforcing The Obvious

*"Your body is a symbol of your whole life, of
who you are, and of what your soul is like.
You co-create your physical self through the laws of science, as well as
through the laws of Spirit."*
~ Dr. Christiane Northrup

Well, knock me down!

I am once again "getting" – for the millionth time – and accepting – for maybe the third time – that it's equally about the irrefutable science of calories in and calories out AND the touchy-feely stuff.

That resistance to counting my calories is starting to slip away. I'd done it faithfully through the good, the bad, and the ugly...like when we went out for sushi, and for dessert we split a tempura chocolate with ice cream and that, along with two glasses of wine, put me well over the edge. But I can see it now!

My effort brings me joy! My acceptance is what brings me joy!

So to recap: I obviously had been eating too much because I gained weight...then I put the brakes on just enough to maintain. Now, it was time to let it go.

It IS Love

As I approached the last Living Lighter class, I didn't expect a loss, but was okay with it. I learned a lot and signed up to take the class again for twelve more weeks. I spent several days being consciously in love with my body and my self, and it sure feels better than being at war. And I noticed several things: I felt free and powerful, my husband was more affectionate, I was more affectionate, I smiled a lot, even at strangers, and it was a relief that I could still feel that way.

At the beginning, I'd written:

"The idea of losing the weight I have regained feels like a much bigger burden than having lost the original 55 pounds. One thing I know for sure is that I don't want to give up. And at the very same time, I know that I can't and don't want to view this as a struggle...as a fight to be fought. Because if I do, that's exactly what I'll get. A fight. A battle. A struggle.

"In the time since I reached that new low on the scale, I have very much been aware that I am on the quest for the sweet spot – that balance between a healthy body weight (and image) and self-acceptance right now. It's elusive. Kind of like love. The harder you look for it, the harder it becomes to find. Actually, it's not 'kind of like love.' It IS love."

After twelve weeks, I haven't found the sweet spot, but I did find self-acceptance. A little.

From Smarties To Nitric Oxide

It's time for some accountability.

On the way home from the final Living Lighter class, I stopped at the store and bought, among other things, a bag of Goldfish crackers and a small bag of Smarties. Why? I am not exactly sure. I think I wanted to test myself but I also think I was engaging in a little magical thinking; "eating this won't count."

Upon arriving home, I ate most of the Goldfish. Then I squirted some dish soap into the bag and threw it in the garbage. Then I ate a lot of Smarties...maybe a third of the bag. I ate more Smarties later in the day, and finished them the next day.

The day I polished off the Smarties, I decided (again) to let go of my resistance to logging my calories. Though I didn't realize it at the time, it was also the day I started to feel more in love with my body.

While reading Dr. Christiane Northrup's book *The Secret Pleasures of Menopause,* this jumped out at me: "The electromagnetic field around your heart (which is the center of your emotions) is a hundred times more powerful than the electromagnetic field of your brain (the center of your thoughts). This means that no matter what you think, what you feel always wins!"

Ah-HA! I hadn't been *feeling* the love, the confidence, the Wow. I'd been *thinking* about it, *hoping* for it, but I wasn't feeling it because how can I feel Wow when I also feel disgust, fear, and shame?

I'm not sure how or why, but I finally let go of the disgust, fear and shame, and actually *felt* the Wow!

It's the difference between thinking positive thoughts, and actually feeling them. Do you know the difference? It's like the difference between thinking about love and feeling it – that honest-to-God physical and emotional yee-haw-I-feel-giddy thing.

Dr. Northrup also discusses nitric oxide (not to be confused with nitrous oxide, or "laughing gas," which is what dentists use). Although, she does call nitric oxide "the happy molecule" and explains that it exists in the lining of our blood vessels.

She explains:

"When nitric oxide is produced, through meditation, exercise, and glorious sex, the smooth muscles in your blood vessels relax. This allows life-nurturing oxygen to be circulated throughout the body, especially to the heart and the brain. Although you might not have known what it was called, you do know about nitric oxide – increasing the quantity and flow of it is the mechanism used in nitroglycerin and in erectile dysfunction drugs like Viagra....

"This is a beautiful, natural mechanism that we need only enhance. I'm not talking about something that numbs the pain, like alcohol or a recreational drug (or food). Increasing your nitric oxide levels requires simply increasing the joy in your life – through pleasurable pursuits of any kind. There are many effective ways to raise our nitric oxide levels."

Dr. Northrup wrote that any activity that enhances the mind-body connection, such as meditation, breathing deeply and rhythmically, practicing yoga, and having sex raises nitric oxide levels in the body.

Now I have more science (remember neural plasticity?) to back up the woo-woo stuff.

My Treasure

Some would say that the Living Lighter class "didn't work" for me because I "only lost two pounds" in twelve weeks (my goal had been to lose six pounds). But I have, indeed, met a different kind of goal. I recovered my treasure.

Back at the beginning of this story and this journey, I mentioned a quote from Joseph Campbell: *"It is by going down into the abyss that we recover the treasures of life. Where you stumble, there lies your treasure."*

I spent a lot of time in the abyss and I always had faith – even when it didn't seem like it – that I would stumble and find my treasure. My treasure is self-acceptance. Heading into my second twelve weeks of Living Lighter, I feel self-acceptance 100%.

More importantly, I learned how to access my treasure more easily and that is key…because I am smart enough to know that I won't *feel* self-acceptance 24/7/365.

I am a human being, after all.

A Meeting With My Evil Twins

I thought it would be a good idea to have a meeting with some of my Evil Twins before the next Living Lighter class starts. They wanted it, I needed it. Overall, I think it went better than similar meetings in the past, but still, it wasn't great. Resistant Karen was the most vocal, and really, she is quite a handful. When she's around, not only am I not productive, I find myself shutting myself off to positive ways of being.

I did notice, however, that during the meeting Wow wasn't too far away – I was aware of it and I remembered how it felt, but I wasn't actually feeling it.

It was like I wanted to test the Wow. Before I went to bed, I sensed that the test was over and I'd passed, but not with flying colors. I meditated briefly using my self-hypnosis script and I was able to smile, because even though I didn't have it memorized verbatim, I remembered the key points:

- I breathe in patience, consistency, and clarity
- I breathe out impatience, inconsistency, and confusion
- I am clear about who I am, what I want, and my commitment to myself. My effort brings me joy.

The next day, in response to a friend mentioning the need to rebuild her self-esteem and find herself again, I wrote: "I know for me, finding Karen is all about that wonderful self-love and acceptance, and just feeling that essence that is uniquely me. Just writing this is making me feel the 'Wow' in my heart."

And it really did. I could tell the Evil Twins had backed off. I have this powerful image of them looking at me with new-found respect, saying amongst themselves, "I guess we can't mess with her like we used to."

The Flash Bulb Of (Self) Love

The day before the second Living Lighter series began I felt cranky and annoyed. My focus and awareness had gone out the window in the week prior, and that meant I was not in love with my body, and that meant I hadn't been eating cleanly, and that meant...what?

I had a feeling that I'd undone the two-pound loss, and I grit my teeth, trying not to let negativity overtake me. I'm breathing, I'm remembering my meditation, I'm thinking about nitric oxide, I'm trying to feel the love in and around my heart.

I love myself...I am okay the way I am...I don't need to be like anyone else...I can be happy no matter what...I have worth...I am walking the right path for me...it's okay to be me...blah blah blah.

Sometimes it feels like I have to constantly remind myself of all this! Damn it! And even when I remind myself, it's hard to feel it! Then I start to wonder what's wrong with me? Why the hell can't I just feel it all the time? And yet I realize that those self-punishing thoughts are counterproductive. I understand I have to keep my guard up, but I'm also angry that I have to keep my guard up.

After kickboxing one morning, a friend and I talked about this, and she observed something about me and put it in a way that gave me a different perspective. She said I am like a flash bulb – I have flashes of self-love, and then the bulb goes dark.

"Trust me," she added, "I give myself the self-love talk every morning in the mirror."

This friend always struck me as someone who is supremely self-confident. She's the kind of person who lights up a room when she walks in, and no, she's not a phony-baloney. She's the real deal. I've admired this about her since we first met. She's the kind of person you want to be around and you think, "I want some of what she's got."

She cultivates and nurtures this in herself every day, and she doesn't see it as keeping her guard up, but as a natural, self-loving part of her day.

Part II: As Long As It Needs To Take....

May 2009

"You cannot struggle to joy.
Struggle and joy are not
on the same channel.
You joy your way to joy." ~ Abraham

Living Lighter, Round Two

I went into the second twelve-week session of Living Lighter with a different purpose and attitude. The first time around I was coming from a place of pain and hurt: desperate, full of dread, focused on being fat. I didn't have the perspective that I do now. This time around, I want to focus on acceptance and health.

My goals for the second twelve weeks:

- To define myself by who I am and what I do, not by a number on the scale or the size of my clothes
- To focus on making choices that serve me
- To give myself the self-love talk at least once a day
- To remind myself regularly that right this minute, I can be okay and happy
- To not punish myself when I am not perfect

I've been thinking about why I have self-esteem issues, and it's clear to me that many of the female role models in my life have the same issues, even if it's not apparent on the surface. They've had a hard time accepting themselves, and they are also hard on themselves.

In the past, I'd looked at it more like "this or that happened" or "this or that was said to me" and I internalized it. But now I see it as something that got passed down through generations. This doesn't mean I'm destined to have the same issues. I'm now more aware of them, and more aware of where they came from. So now, I can change it.

Thanks, Mom

One thing I never wanted this book to be is a place where I bash or blame my parents – or anyone else – for anything. I don't consider myself a victim in any sense of the word, but I am fascinated with the mother-daughter dynamic. I know that relationship can be fraught with unique and intense pain and love at the same time.

So along with realizing I come from a long line of women who may have had a hard time accepting themselves, I wanted to share this...

I attended a women's networking event where the speaker focused on the writings of Joan Anderson, author of *A Year by the Sea*, among other books. The idea was that we are all "unfinished women" who generally give way more than we take, and do more for others than for ourselves. We're wives, mothers, daughters, sisters, business owners, caretakers, and so on.

This is something to which I've never really related. In fact, sometimes I wonder if there's something wrong with me because I'm not "stressed out" and I tend to have too much time on my hands.

As I listened to the speaker talk about how women rarely take time for themselves, and how they're always doing for others, I realized that my mother was an excellent role model for *not* being one of those women. Don't get me wrong: she was and is a busy woman and she took good care of me. She also worked either full or part time; went back to college when I was in high school and graduated with high honors; was involved in the community; played bridge with her friends; and had an active life. But she also took time for herself. There was never any sense of being a stressed out martyr. She taught me that it was all about choices.

For my mother, taking time for herself meant traveling, either alone, with my stepfather, or with friends. When I was in my early twenties, she saved some money, sold her house, quit her job, and traveled around the world for about a year. Go, Mom!

Along with modeling the idea that women need to take time for themselves, she also instilled in me the confidence to travel any time, anywhere. I remember flying by myself from Missouri to New York when I was six, and taking a three-hour train trip by myself when I was twelve to visit my dad. When I got my driver's license at sixteen, there was no question I'd be able to drive myself anywhere! There is such freedom in having the confidence to travel, and my mother set me free in that way!

As I said, I used to feel guilty because I'm not one of those women always doing, doing, doing. But now, I'm much more grateful than guilty. Thanks, Mom.

I Have Wow Now

I mentioned approaching the second round of Living Lighter with different purpose and attitude – relaxed and happy instead of defensive and desperate. Thank God! Because it feels so much better this way!

In Round One, I equated committing to the process with suffering, so I resisted committing.

In Round Two, I equate commitment as being gentle with myself; thinking about my choices before I make them; using the online calorie tracker as a helpful tool to make sure I'm on track and not as a rigid all-or-nothing, I'm-a-failure-if-I-miss-a-day torture chamber.

That said, there is still some work to be done.

At the start of week two, Amy asked what negative feelings or faulty thoughts I might have this time around, and I realized that I might not want it bad enough..."it" being weight loss.

We went through the "feel an emotion that leads to a faulty thought, then turn it around" exercise.

What feeling leads me to think "I might not want it bad enough?" Could it be fear? On the surface, no, but deeper down, I suppose it could still be a defense. If I don't want it, then I can't fail...but even in processing that idea, I felt an overwhelming sense of "yes, I can!" Fail, that is.

How does this faulty thought serve me? It gives me permission to eat more than I need in those moments when I may be wavering. It's also a control issue. If I don't want it, then I am in control. If I want it, but can't get it, then it must be out of my control.

How would my life be different if I never believed this thought again? If I didn't believe "I don't want it bad enough," nothing would hold me back!

Turn it around. For me, the opposite of "I don't want it bad enough" is "I have Wow now."

Can't vs. Won't:
Revisiting Psychological Uneasiness

I know I've had moments when I truly felt "I can't." I lacked awareness and mindless eating was the norm. Now that I'm aware, mindless eating is pretty much impossible. So when I make a choice that doesn't serve me, it's not about "I can't" but rather "I can, but I don't want to" or "I won't." I understand that on the surface there's power in having made a conscious choice, but when it comes to my health there's no power in making a bad choice *on purpose*.

So let's talk about responsibility. What does it really mean to be responsible? In simple terms, responsibility = the ability to respond. If you take it a step further, responsibility = the ability to respond in a powerful and positive way.

What do I gain by being irresponsible with my eating habits? Weight. I gain weight. Ha-ha. But seriously, while I've come a long way in the emotional overeating department, I'm not where I'd ultimately like to be. Stay tuned for a powerful chapter on that subject.

Sometimes, I give in to psychological uneasiness. After a rather upsetting day recently, I felt fragile and in need of comforting. I chose to comfort myself with food.

The good news is I feel no shame over it.

Ultimately, I AM Where I Want To Be

When the book *The Secret* first came out, I was all over it. The Law of Attraction wasn't new, but *The Secret* made it accessible and reminded us about it at a time when we really seemed to needed it. The Law of Attraction states that like begets like, scientifically, spiritually, physically, mentally, emotionally…in every way.

I imagined that it was the magic answer I had been looking for. Then somewhere along the way, without realizing it, I let skepticism, doubt, and negativity creep back in…specifically regarding how I view my body.

A friend had been reading *The Secret* in fits and starts, and one night, she picked it up again and randomly opened to the chapter "The Secret and Our Bodies." After reading it, she wanted to challenge herself to erase all negative thoughts about her body, her exercise, her eating, and thoughts about her "diet."

"The definition of the perfect weight is the weight that feels good for you. No one else's opinion counts. It is the weight that feels good to you."

"As you think perfect thoughts, as you feel good about YOU, you are on the frequency of your perfect weight, and you are summoning perfection."

My friend reminded me that PERFECTION IS DEFINED BY WHAT FEELS GOOD TO YOU. Not by society, not by *Vogue*, not by *Cosmo*, not by *Shape,* not by your friends, not by your family. Only you define it!

And remember: it's not good enough to just say it. You must believe it.

Although I didn't know it when I first started, this is exactly where I'm going with this book. Here's that "powerful chapter" I mentioned earlier.

When I first started writing this book, the title I chose was *Why Weight: One Woman's Journey from Struggle to Acceptance* and it was chosen for a reason. I know that if I view this as a struggle, then that's what it will be. I have friends who talk about weight loss as a battle to be fought, as war! I have a visceral reaction when I hear that. I don't want to struggle! I don't want to fight! I'm a lover, not a fighter!

But as I said, somewhere along the way I forgot. I struggled. I AM ultimately where I want to be.

The Awed Silence Of Self-Acceptance

Melancholy is two parts sad and one part sweet. I accept melancholy. A few weeks into my second round of Living Lighter, it rained for nearly a solid week, so I'm sure that played a role in how I felt. Also, I stepped on the scale for the first time in several weeks and my weight was the same. For a moment, I was disappointed, but then I remembered that my clothes fit me better than they did a month ago, I feel better – physically and emotionally – and, what the hell, it's just a number. The scale has lost its power over me.

I think this might also be the awed silence of self-acceptance. The voices in my head had been pretty quiet, and I wasn't used to all that silence. It was a little scary – but just a little. I might have been mourning the loss of that self that didn't know self-acceptance. She served me in some ways over the years, and held me back in other ways. Realizing she was gone, I guess it was natural to feel a little melancholy.

But I also felt something I hadn't felt before...at least not that I can recall. Perhaps, up till this point, I'd been "faking it till I make it." And now, I'm not faking it anymore.

My Name Is Karen...

Much of this has been about the emotional component of being overweight, and I have come a long way, baby, in that regard. But you know what? I thought loving and accepting myself would be enough for the weight to just fall right off me, as if I'd taken a magic pill! But it isn't, and it hasn't.

What's interesting is I am able to smile about it. I'm not desperate. I'm not frustrated. I'm not distraught. I'm not angry. I still love and accept myself!

So what's the deal? Why is the weight hanging on?

My name is Karen, and I'm addicted to sugar. Not only do I admit it, I accept it.

You'd think that I would have crossed this bridge already. I think I've known about the addiction, but I've been deeply in denial. Admitting to any sort of addiction is hard for me because I was brought up to believe that addiction is either a personality defect or a cop out.

In my mind, however, not all sugar is created equal. I have specific cravings and certain sugary, starchy foods (and wine) will definitely "set me off" on a binge. I don't think of myself as really liking sweet foods – in fact, I'm often turned off by food or drink that is overly sweet – but when I'm craving sugar and starch, these are my "go to" choices in no particular order:

- Smartfood popcorn or kettlecorn

- Smarties
- Goldfish crackers
- Any chocolate/peanut butter item
- Potato chips
- Chex Mix
- Homemade chocolate chip cookies
- Croutons
- Wine

If any of these items are in the house, it's almost impossible to control myself while eating them, especially if I'm hungry. Ice cream, tortilla chips, cake, muffins, dark chocolate, pretzels, beer or any other type of alcohol? No problem. Those items are "safe."

My goal is to not eat any food that has more than seven grams of sugar per serving and, as I've said before, to avoid "white" foods – bread, sugar, pasta, potatoes, rice, etc. I am also researching and seeking out the latest information about food and sugar addiction.

First up on my reading list is *The End of Overeating* by Dr. David A. Kessler. In it, he explains how "our bodies and minds are changed when we eat foods that contain sugar, fat and salt and how food manufacturers manipulate these ingredients to stimulate our appetites."

Author Martha Beck also has written a book called *The Four Day Win: End your Diet War and Achieve Thinner Peace*, which outlines some fascinating research about the brain and how to train it, and your body, to get thin.

So now it's time to deal with this physiological/biological issue of sugar addiction. The good news is that emotionally I am prepared and healthy!

Karen's Rules Of Trigger Food Disengagement

In his book *The End of Overeating*, Dr. David Kessler
recommends having "rules of disengagement" that take control
away from the trigger foods and place it squarely back with
oneself. So without further delay, here are my Rules of Trigger
Food Disengagement (so far):

I refuse foods I can't control (trigger foods).

I limit the amount of time I am exposed to trigger foods.

I remember what's at stake.

I don't stop. I walk on by. I turn my attention elsewhere.

I actively resist when necessary.

I use the thought-stopping technique. When I experience a
trigger, I switch off the associated thought immediately. No
debates. No maybes.

I use the counter-conditioning technique. As I experience a
trigger, I immediately associate it with a negative consequence.
"If I eat that, I will feel awful." I undercut the reward value of
the trigger.

I imagine myself in the familiar scenario of purchasing trigger
foods. Then I imagine the aftermath: How does my body feel
when I eat a whole bag of Goldfish crackers? What effect will it

have on the scale? What effect will it have on my body? How will I feel emotionally?

I talk down the urge:

- "Eating that will satisfy me only temporarily."
- "Eating that will keep me trapped in a vicious sugar cycle."
- "Eating that will make me feel bad, both emotionally and physically."
- "I'll be happier in the long run if I don't eat that."
- "I'll weigh less if I don't eat that."

It Takes As Long As It Needs To Take

Constantly thinking about losing weight is making me crazy. It exhaust me. I've been thinking about it in one way or another for almost 40 years! I just want to take a break and enjoy myself. I'm tired of being vigilant and I wonder if it's really necessary?

It's been slow going, but I think I' finally getting to that sweet spot. First came the "self-acceptance right now" even though I am 20-plus pounds heavier than I was at my lowest weight in 2006. From that came a willingness to seek out information and knowledge I might not already have. I am joyfully embracing "healthy eating" and it doesn't feel like a struggle. And if the scale is any indication, my body is releasing the weight once again...*new* weight, not the same five pounds I'd been playing with for months and months and months and MONTHS!

This Is What I'm Talkin' About

I've upped my protein for breakfast and lunch, and I've been consistent with it. Every day. Yeah me...Miss Anti-Consistency.

But guess what? I love how eating 60 to 70 grams of protein before 2:00 p.m. every day makes me feel, so why stop?

In case you're wondering what 60 to 70 grams of protein looks like, here you go:

- Breakfast: Oatmeal with protein powder and an egg mixed in before cooking, OR two eggs, two turkey sausage breakfast links, and two Kashi waffles.
- Lunch: Five ounces of tuna, mixed with a variety of fresh veggies and served on whole-grain pita with a slice of melted cheddar.
- Snack: Non-fat Greek yogurt with fresh peach slices OR low fat cottage cheese with fresh pineapple chunks.

Please note, this is NOT a low-carb diet.

I used to be afraid to consume too many calories in the first part of the day because I thought I wouldn't have enough for later, which is when my hunger kicks in. Besides, it wasn't like I was ever starving in the morning. But the fact is, when I eat more protein for breakfast and lunch, I don't *need or want* to eat a lot later in the day!

But one afternoon, there was an exception. I felt rather unfocused, distracted, and yes, hungry...even after eating a protein-packed breakfast and lunch. Momentarily, I panicked and felt annoyed, which was accompanied by fleeting thoughts:

Maybe I'll just go ahead and eat whatever! What the heck? Could it be that this is just one more stupid plan that won't work? That I am a freaking loser who's hungry when she shouldn't be?

Of course I'm not. I'm so not going there. The reason I felt hungry was I'd had some wine the day before and that extra sugar was making itself known to me. It's simple chemistry and biology, nothing more. And with that, I gritted my teeth, ate ten almonds, and forgot about it until dinnertime.

This Is What Peace Feels Like

I was going to call this a minor accomplishment, but it is, in fact, a rather major victory.

Tim went out of town for the first time since I started eating more protein for breakfast and lunch. In the past, Tim being out of town meant I wouldn't take care of myself, and that usually meant I wouldn't make myself dinner. I'd meander up and down the grocery store aisles looking for foods on which to binge – like Smarties or Goldfish crackers and perhaps a couple glasses of wine to wash it all down. My sugar drugs of choice.

None of that happened. This afternoon, I went to the store and bought non-binge-inducing foods like fresh raspberries, spinach, Kashi waffles, Greek yogurt, and tuna. I went to kickboxing class at 7:15 p.m. after making myself a light dinner.

I'd be lying if I said I didn't think about getting some wine, and that I didn't look at the Goldfish crackers about a second longer than necessary as I walked past the cracker and cookie aisle. I had a couple "I've been so good a little something won't hurt" thoughts. But those thoughts weren't like clanging cymbals in my head. They were just…thoughts.

As I finished my light supper, I thought, "Oh, this isn't going to be enough. I still feel a little hungry. How am I going to feel after I kickbox?" I decided to worry about it later. I brushed my teeth (because no one likes a kickboxing partner with bad breath) and voila! Hunger gone! It wasn't real.

I kickboxed for 45 minutes, came home, and took a shower. I knew my raspberries were waiting for me, and a cup of chamomile tea. I wasn't hungry. I wasn't annoyed. I wasn't frantic. I wasn't struggling, holding myself back at all costs from jumping into the abyss. I wasn't craving anything at all. I was truly at peace. My body and my psyche were on the same page.

Temptation

In a recent Living Lighter class, Amy asked, "What is your temptation, and how do you resist?" I knew she wasn't talking about Goldfish crackers or Smarties. She was talking about those behaviors that tempt me away from the path I'm on: the path of self-acceptance and a healthy body weight.

I made a few notes.

"I am tempted to have someone else tell me what to do."

"I am tempted to have someone hold my hand."

"I am tempted to give up control."

And then it came to me...

"I am tempted to be confused."

Being confused serves me because someone else will "take care of it" – "it" being whatever it is I don't want to deal with.

Being confused also *hurts* me because it keeps me stalled, and it's depressing. When I'm confused and want to stick my head in the sand, I don't grow and learn. And that feels bad. And then I want to numb and comfort myself. And the cycle continues.

If confusion didn't exist for me, what would my life look like?

I'd be clear about everything I want and I'd just do it.

I find that when I'm in a good mood, there is no confusion. I'm clear about what I want and I'm not tempted to be confused and stalled. There's no struggle and I make choices that support what I want for myself.

So how do I extract myself from this funk?

I've developed a couple of mantras that I've been repeating:

"Suffering is optional" and "It is my choice to have a good day no matter what."

Did I give in to my temptation? Yes, I did and I spent a little time comforting myself with food. The good news is that I'm still in the habit of getting that protein in, that I took the time to figure out what was tempting me, and that I can turn it around and reverse the stall.

What tempts you? What takes your attention away from the path you're on? The temptation to be distracted? Confused? Passive? In control? Out of control? The temptation to hide, to cave, or to give up?

In the end, it's about mastering the ability to turn our temptation around and getting right back on the path to living the lives we desire.

Altering My Thoughts

It's amazing to me how quickly negativity can creep back in, even if we only open the door a crack. I went into the Living Lighter class feeling rather negative, even after all my previous realizations about being tempted into confusion. The act of getting clear brought me face-to-face with the scale...which hadn't budged an inch, and so familiar thoughts flooded my mind.

"But I've been so good!"

"Damn. I guess the potato chips and strawberry shortcake on Saturday were a HUGE mistake even though I ate so very healthy the whole rest of the time."

"I am soooo tired of thinking about this."

"I need to let go."

"What is wrong with me?"

So, at class, I dumped all my negative thoughts onto paper with the intent of shredding it as soon as I was done.

Then, quoting authors Esther and Jerry Hicks (who have written extensively about the law of attraction), Amy wrote, *"Moving from a negative 'knowing' to a positive, life-affirming 'realization' takes either a bolt of lightning or a series of successive alterations of thought."*

She asked me what my most negative thought was.

"I am weak."

She then led me through a series of successive alterations to get to the opposite, which I stated as "I am strong enough to do anything." Successive alterations are statements that I believe to be true.

While she explained how the process worked, I had a small "bolt of lightning" thought: I am often surprised when I am viewed in a positive light. I've been known to say things like "Wow, she really likes me" or "I guess I made a good impression" or "I can't believe I've made such good friends." It's often a revelation to me when I'm accepted or liked or included, and I'm often surprised at my level of strength and fitness because it wasn't all that long ago that I couldn't walk up a hill without having to take a break.

But back to the successive alterations that take me from "I am weak" to "I am strong enough to do anything."

- There are times when I am NOT weak.
- I feel strong when I do things that support me.
- When I feel strong, I am in control.
- That out-of-control person is not who I am.
- I may have moments of weakness but my commitment remains strong.
- It is possible to believe that I am strong, and it is also helpful to believe it.
- The number on the scale is not an indicator of my strength.
- I am strong whether or not I feel that I am.

- So, the truth is, I am strong enough to do anything.

This exercise got me thinking about the damn scale. I've gone back and forth about whether or not weighing myself is good for me. I have moments when the number is nothing more than an objective measure of one aspect of my physical self, and moments when it's an indication that I am a weak, unmotivated, and undisciplined slacker.

So I had to ask myself whether weighing myself moves me towards strength or weakness. Are there other less painful ways to gauge my strength and progress?

How my clothes fit and how I feel are good gauges, as are monitoring my calorie intake and my moods.

So, for the time being, the scale goes in the closet.

Relax. Just Do It.

There's a school of thought that suggests people should eat as much as they want in their quest for healthy weight loss. The theory is that if we let ourselves have whatever we want, when we want it, maybe we won't want it as much as we think we do.

What often trips me up is the fact that I lost 55 pounds. So I can't wrap my mind around the idea of eating what I want because I view that as eating the way I might have before I lost that weight. Does that make sense?

Sometimes I think I just need to let go of everything. All of it. I can't go back to the old ways of being and eating because I am not that person. It's not who I am.

This leads me to a faulty thought I've had for a long time: "I need to be in tight, strict control at all times because I can't trust myself."

I think part of this has to do with the fact that I *think* I lost 55 pounds by being in tight, strict control all of the time, even though I don't remember it being that way.

So what is the opposite? How do I want to think instead?

How about, "I trust myself to do what supports my health and I can relax because I know it, deep within myself"?

How do successive alterations come into play?

- I can't trust myself so I must be in strict control at all times. I can't relax! I must be vigilant!
- When I am not vigilant, I am out of control and I become angry with myself.
- There are times when I'm not in strict control, BUT not wildly out of control either.
- There are times when I trust myself.
- When I allow myself to feel good, I trust myself.
- When I accept myself, I trust myself.
- It is possible to believe that I can just relax and trust myself, and it's also *helpful* to believe it.
- I CAN trust myself AND relax, whether or not I feel it.
- So, the truth is, I trust myself to do what supports my health and I can relax now because I *know* it, deep within myself.

A friend who has reached her goal weight and maintained wrote:

"It's such a tricky balance, isn't it? I believe that the one reason I have had positive results this time around is that I have trusted myself more than ever. And yet I know that part of me is still wanting to play 'getting away with it' games and so I have to have a certain level of vigilance. For example, I have not 'allowed' myself to just 'go for it' and eat things that have triggered me in the past because I just don't trust that I can eat a small amount and feel satisfied. Some things, especially desserts, I can be okay with a small taste and actually feel satisfied, but other things – mostly carb-y comfort foods, not yet."

The "getting away with it" game struck a chord with me. I've played it many times. But my thinking has shifted a bit. I know I can't have certain foods in the house, but I now feel "I don't eat those any more…that's not who I am." So those foods aren't on my radar – at least, not right now. It's not like I really want to eat them and I'm holding myself back with white knuckles.

On the other hand, there are foods that are perfectly fine but which I still associate with guilt and "being bad." I don't binge on those foods, but I often feel the need to justify eating them. I also feel guilt while eating them.

Being that way hurts me on a psychic level – it hurts my body's psyche to feel guilt rather than enjoying my food. Not trusting myself also hurts my body's psyche. So the intent with which I eat something is just as important – if not *more* important – than what I am eating.

Continually Learning My Lessons, Part I

It always amazes me how a seemingly insignificant stream of events can lead to learning a rather significant lesson.

My Dad came to visit and I invited him to watch me kickbox. He was duly impressed. Afterward, he said, "You should keep your elbows in closer to your sides." He quickly added, "It was towards the end of class...you were probably tired."

You have to understand, he didn't say it in a critical or judgmental tone; it was said in a rather kindly way.

But I bristled. I thought, "He always finds something to criticize...what the hell...he has a lot of nerve to criticize me. I'd like to see him get up there and train like I did for two hours!"

But I also knew he was right.

In the car on the way home, I said – in a mostly neutral tone of voice – that he has a tendency to find something to criticize and I reminded him of several times that he'd done so.

We didn't argue or have harsh words; it was sort of humorous and light. One thing you have to realize is I didn't grow up with my Dad. He and my mother divorced when I was three, but I saw him often and idolized him for the longest time. I found it hard to be mad at him for anything. It's only been in the last ten years or so that I think our relationship has become more of a "normal" adult father/daughter relationship. I notice a widening divide in how we think socially and politically, and I am more apt to say what I think. It's a healthier relationship.

But back to his comment about my elbows…

It stayed with me and I thought about the various ways I might have responded instead. I could have just said, "Gee, you're right, Dad…that's something I have to work on." Later, I told him my thoughts. I also told him about "soft eyes," and how I've been working on having soft eyes for both myself and for others.

The more I thought about it, the more I thought about how good it feels to forgive myself for my imperfections, and how, when I feel less critical of myself, I am less critical of others. I also thought about how parents in general are able to elicit bristly responses in their children – especially when trying to avoid it – and how, perhaps, the parents might be critical of themselves.

In the end, I think it boils down to being disappointed when our parents aren't perfect, even though we know they can't be or shouldn't be. That got me thinking about the times in my life when I've been harsh or critical, and in hindsight, that felt "icky."

Over the years I've had what seemed like all-consuming "issues" with various members of my family. I remember that all I wanted to do was spew-spew-spew to anyone who would listen. Being critical, judgmental and right is what was modeled in my family, so I didn't know any other way of being, even though I didn't like being that way! I used to think there was something wrong with me because I hate conflict and tension and I tend not to know how to be a logical, critical (in a positive way) thinker.

Now I understand that it just doesn't jibe with who I am.

And in the process of writing this, I figured something out. In those years when I was spewing my venom, I was either afraid to be myself or I didn't know how. And in my confusion, I punished myself with food.

It's interesting for me to see my evolution from "woman who has issues" to "woman who is pretty much okay with everything"…to observe my own reactions, to be more objective and say "Oh, look at that – you bristled" or "Cool, you didn't let your buttons get pushed that time." It's not like we change overnight or in a linear fashion. We bump along, sometimes revisiting old stuff. But over time, we find ourselves making some progress.

Continually Learning My Lessons, Part II

Forgive yourself for everything you didn't know in the past. Don't waste any of your precious energy beating up yourself or anyone else. Your power to change your life is in the present, regardless of your past.
~ Dr. Christiane Northrup

I still have a lot of work to do.

I recently put myself in a situation that I knew would be difficult, based on many years of previous experience. I set some specific goals: no raised voices and no tears. I even made a pact with myself. In order to meet these goals I vowed that I would:

- avoid subjects that I know are "button pushing" subjects
- change the subject tactfully if "button pushing" topics came up
- take deep breaths and soften my eyes when feeling myself wanting to react
- remember the healthy boundaries I have set in the past, boundaries that protect
- be loving
- avoid having an agenda
- enjoy myself
- be myself

The results were mixed.

On the positive side, there were no raised voices and no tears; I avoided "button pushing," I avoided outwardly reacting, and I banished my agenda. I am proud of myself for that because it used to be that I seemingly had no control over my emotions in this particular situation.

On the negative side, I wasn't able to set healthy boundaries and that resulted in feeling powerless and impotent and so I reacted inwardly. I was NOT myself because previous experience shows that I need to keep my guard up. There are times when I can relax, but that can change quickly. I went from feeling mildly frustrated and annoyed to feeling burning, boiling rage. It brings me to tears just thinking about it now, days later.

I tried so hard to avoid outward conflict that I created huge amounts of it within. In hindsight, my goal should have been "create harmony" not "avoid conflict."

Here I thought I was doing a good thing by avoiding the conflict, but what I really did was resist a hard place, a difficult time, and so I lost an opportunity to grow. I lost an opportunity to be authentically me. Maybe I'm still not exactly sure what that means.

The point of writing this is to get to the next point. In the last chapter I wrote:

"Over the years I've had what seemed like all-consuming 'issues' with various members of my family. I remember that all I wanted to do was spew spew spew to anyone who would listen. Being critical, judgmental and right is what was modeled in my family so I didn't know any other way of being, even though I didn't like being that

way! I used to think there was something wrong with me because I hate conflict and tension and I tend not to know how to be a logical, critical (in a positive way) thinker. Now I understand that it just doesn't jibe with who I am. And in the process of writing this, I figured something out: in those years when I was spewing my venom, I was either afraid to be myself, or I didn't know how. And so I punished myself with food."

So the next piece of the puzzle is realizing that putting up and shutting up is not the opposite of spewing venom. It's not being me. And it can have the same result: abusing myself with food. As I left that situation I stopped to get gas. I also got a bag of Cheez-Its and a bag of peanut butter M&Ms. I'm not even going to talk about being "good" and "bad" but suffice it to say that up until that moment, I had reached a very nice Zen place as it concerns food.

I knew as I was purchasing this stuff that I was doing it to both comfort and abuse myself. It wasn't a mindless binge, something that I "woke up" from after the fact. I went into it with my eyes wide open. And I even remembered what I had written and figured "what the hell."

I Poured A Bottle of Wine Down The Drain

I've said it several times: "In the end, it takes as long as it needs to take." Here's another example of that.

I've been in the habit of drinking wine almost every night. This is a habit I've had on and off for years, and I'm starting to see a connection to other things that are going on in my life...things that I don't like.

First and most obviously are bloat and apparent weight gain (I say "apparent" because I'm not weighing myself, but I know my body oh-so-well). Secondly, I'd noticed lethargy and an overall dull feeling (sort of depressed, but not really). Thirdly, I'd noticed achy joints. I'm not sure why, but instinct tells me that it's the wine making me ache.

Over the years, I've gone back and forth between being an "every day" drinker and not drinking much at all. There have been times when I've questioned whether or not I might be an alcoholic. I don't think I am – I think it's related more to the sugar in the wine – but at the same time, the whole thing makes me defensive because of my family history and their dysfunction around alcohol (it's that "all or nothing" thing).

All I know is if there's wine in the house, I'll drink it.

One night, as I lay in bed, watching television and drinking too much wine, I thought about how this does not serve me. In fact, I almost felt like a slave to it. I'd also noticed feeling almost obligated to drink...like it's just expected. I'd never felt that way before.

So I decided to stop buying wine to have around the house "just in case." In fact, I took the last bottle in the house and poured it down the kitchen sink. I needed to give myself a break.

This ties into something else that had been weighing on me (and, yes, I AM meant to live lighter!): being distracted.

I allow myself to become distracted by so many things, and yes, I see that wine drinking as a distraction. I lose my focus easily. Sometimes I chalk it up to being "creative" but in fact I'm finding distraction to be somewhat destructive. So along with no wine in the house, I challenge myself to do one thing at a time, and to focus on that one thing, for at least 15 minutes at a time.

Old patterns run deep. There's that little voice inside that tells me that I'd be judged, not for wanting to make my life better, but for not having had a better life in the first place. But what I'm realizing is that instead of all these ideas that there must be something wrong with me – that I am bad – I'm coming at it from a place of acceptance. And that's what this journey has been about for me: making better decisions for myself because I love and accept Me, not because I loathe Me.

Tending Towards Fat

You know when you set your mind to something, or you have an "ah-ha" moment, and then all of a sudden you start noticing things you wouldn't have noticed before? Like the Universe is trying to tell you something?

After pouring that bottle of wine down the drain, I noticed all kinds of things. First was this quote by Dr. Christiane Northrup:

"If you don't heed the messages from your body the first time they're delivered, you'll get hit with a bigger hammer the next time. A delay or denial requires you body to speak louder and louder to get your attention. The purpose of emotions, regardless of what they are, is to help you feel and participate fully in your own life. Stop and experience them! Then change your behavior accordingly."

Wine was the hammer. And my body was speaking louder.

Then Tim and I spent a week in Nova Scotia to celebrate our 12th anniversary. Although we both brought our laptop computers with us, I vowed that I wouldn't spend needless time distracting myself on the Internet. I wanted to get into the habit of doing one thing at a time…focusing on one thing at a time…without feeling the need to check email, check Facebook, listen to voicemail, or whatever else seemed attractive at the time.

I noticed things in Nova Scotia. People drive more slowly and are much more aware of - and friendly to - pedestrians, especially in Halifax. There's also a relaxed pace to eating in restaurants. I was really struck by how food is prepared, portioned, and served. We easily spent two hours at dinner every evening, and not just in fancy restaurants. The servers and staff were attentive, but not overbearing and not in a rush to get us out. Serving sizes were appropriate. It was pleasant. It's something I've noticed in other countries. It's something I strive to do at home and when eating out, though I've never really been successful. Experiencing all this again in my new frame of mind made a big impact.

While there, Tim and I went on a three-hour hike along some of the most spectacular shoreline in the world. Afterward, we stopped for lunch at a local deli. Tim said he wasn't that hungry. I was ravenous. We got a couple of wrap sandwiches and Tim said, "Boy, these things are huge" and that he might not be able to eat all of his.

Inside, I was fuming. Not only did I think could eat all of mine, I also knew I'd probably still be hungry afterward. In fact, I was angry that I was hungry in the first place and Tim wasn't. I was angry because our dinner reservations weren't until 7:30 p.m. and I didn't want to appear like a piggy after eating my "huge" sandwich. I was angry because I felt like eating out of control.

I know myself well enough to know that when I feel like this, it's usually hormonal, and that was certainly the case this time. I forgave myself a little, but still felt like I'd taken several steps backward.

What's interesting is that, in the end, I didn't finish the whole sandwich – mostly because I didn't want to eat more than Tim did – and I was able to wait for dinner without dying of hunger. But I was still angry about it.

After my anger subsided, I remembered reading an article about the habits of naturally thin people and those who tend towards fat.

My husband is a naturally thin person and I've often been amazed at his relationship with food. He chews slowly, can deal with being hungry, and would rather wait for a meal than snack (that's not to say that he doesn't have snacks, but not within an hour of a planned meal). Because he eats slowly, his brain cues him when he's had enough to eat. He rarely gets "stuffed." He doesn't eat mindlessly. For example, if he wants chips and salsa, he takes out a portion of chips and puts it in a bowl with a little salsa on the side. Or he can eat a small piece of chocolate and leave it at that.

There's a book titled *Act Thin, Be Thin* by Howard Richman. The book outlines 65 behaviors that people who struggle with their weight tend to have. It shows how our behavior patterns influence our eating habits. Among those patterns are:

- Pushing away compliments
- Skipping meals
- Eating while doing other activities
- Attempting to do more than one thing at a time
- Interrupting people
- Fidgeting
- Perfectionism

Richman says that thin people tend to be focused, inner directed, concentrated, linear thinkers/speakers, listeners, patient, tenacious, all about process, planners for gratification, aware of themselves, calm, preferential to solitude, emotionally open, and methodical.

Those of us who tend to be fat are distracted, outer-directed, diffuse, attentive to many things, and have modular thought/speech. We are talkers, impatient, vacillating, all about the goal, in need of instant gratification, aware of others and prefer company, but are emotionally guarded, and spontaneous.

Thin...Fat
Focused...Distracted
Inner-directed...Outer directed
Concentrated...Diffused
Attention on one thing...Attention on many things
Linear thought/speech...Modular thought/speech
Listens...Talks
Patient...Impatient
Tenacious...Vacillating
Sees the process...Sees the goal
Planned gratification...Instant gratification
Aware of self...Aware of others
Calm...Frantic
Prefers solitude...Prefers company
Emotionally open...Emotionally guarded
Methodical...Spontaneous

With few exceptions, my mind tends toward "fat"...and Tim certainly tends toward "thin." I think I've always known on some level that this is part of my problem. I want to change the "fat tendencies," not because I think they make me a bad person, but because I don't feel good inside when my life trends in the "fat" direction. And my life had been trending that way for a couple of years.

I know the answer lies in setting a goal – something that, until now, I have not wanted to do.

Focusing On A Goal

People who know me well know that I don't like setting goals. The word "goal" has a negative connotation for me. When I hear it or say it, I have a visceral reaction -everything ranging from a big old eye-roll to fear. I am afraid to set goals. How many times do I have to say it?

When I think about this fear, it's rather miraculous that I was able to lose any weight at all in the past, because I know that losing weight requires focusing on a goal and, alas, it appears that I don't know how to focus. Well, that's just bullshit, isn't it?

How does fear creep in?

How many times have I gotten all excited about doing something – not just losing weight, but all kinds of things! – shouted it to the world and then stagnated?

Conversely, how many times have I decided to just stagnate and not have a goal so I don't fail?

The weight that I regained answers that.

I have a friend who has lost 90+ pounds and she just participated in her first figure competition. A figure competition is like bodybuilding, but emphasizes muscle symmetry and tone, versus muscle size. She spent a lot of time training her body, but she also had to train her mind. It was an amazing journey for her…and inspirational for those of us who know her!

A realization had been building for me, and something my friend wrote after the competition brought it front and center: "Never, EVER tell yourself you can't do something. Weight loss is about strengthening our minds and pushing through our fears. YOU CAN!"

I've been afraid and I've been distracting myself from that fear. I need to strengthen my mind and push through my fear. No more distraction! It's time to set a goal!

I know well enough that goals should be SMART: specific, measurable, achievable, realistic, and time-framed. An obvious goal might be "losing X pounds" and then setting up an eating plan, exercising, and weighing myself weekly to work toward the goal.

Instead, however, I decided rather than measuring my weight (which has been problematic for me in the past), I would measure my waist. My goal isn't to spot reduce or anything like that – I realize that doing the right things will result in fat loss and building muscle all over.

I consulted a fitness expert. Should I measure weekly? What kinds of changes should I see? For example, I know that one to two pounds per week is reasonable for weight loss. What should I be shooting for with my waist? Is this a valid measurement?

I decided to aim to lose one-quarter of an inch every two weeks. Based on that, it would take me two months to lose one inch. Ultimately, I need to get my waist measurement under 35 inches, but I'll reassess after two months to determine the next goal.

To achieve my goal. I will:

- Consistently track my food, aiming for no more than 1600 calories per day, focusing on lean protein, fiber, and "good" carbs and fats that keep me satisfied (it's when sugar creeps in that I'm in trouble!)
- Continue kickboxing 4 to 5 times per week, and I will do 30 to 45 minutes of cardio (walking, running, or interval training either outdoors or on the treadmill) one to two times per week.

In my kickboxing classes, we usually do anywhere from 50 to 100 (or more) pushups and 50 to 100 (or more) ab exercises, planks, mountain climbers, jump squats, lunges, etc. I think my exercise is okay. It is food and drink that has really been my issue.

So I guess it's okay to say that there's more than one way to decide if you're making progress toward a goal – if getting on the scale is too much pressure, try measurements, or using a favorite article of clothing as a guide. You know I am all for finding ways that make self-acceptance easier.

What You Resist, Persists

I've been thinking about motivation and how it feels different now than it did a few years ago. Is it a matter of being ready and willing? When I lost 55 pounds, I was on top of the world and the happiest I have ever been. And then apparently I lost that "ready and willing" feeling and gained 20+ pounds.

Why?

I've been trying to answer that question for a long time! And I think there are several answers, from the obvious to the not-so-obvious.

Am I not the same person I was then?

A key theme of this book is moving from struggle to acceptance, moving from being motivated by pain to being motivated by joy and the desire to live lighter in all ways. So why is pain such an effective motivator, and why, when we're happy, do we seem to forget about the goals we made from a place of pain?

The concept of "what you resist, persists" goes like this: if you resist something, you become just like the thing you resist. For example, if you push your left fist into the open palm of your open right hand, your right palm assumes the shape of your fist, unless you make your right palm rigid, and thus, resist the left fist. By resisting, however, we define ourselves in opposition to what we resist, and so we become controlled by what we resist.

As I lay in bed one night, I thought about the resist/persist thing, annoyed because I couldn't sleep. I realized that because I was annoyed, because I wasn't just letting myself feel "I can't sleep" – I couldn't sleep. And the more I just allowed myself to feel it, the sleepier I got, and then I was asleep.

And in the moments before I fell asleep, I had a fleeting thought: I've been struggling against struggling. I don't want to struggle. I want "it" to come easily and naturally. But in my struggle not to struggle, guess what? A struggle is just what I've been getting.

In a moment of pain, I set a goal for myself: lose one inch off my waist in two months. Part of setting the goal involved making some commitments to myself, such as doing (or not doing) certain things that, until that moment, I hadn't been willing to do (or not do). I've kept my promise to myself and it's been rather easy. I'm one millimeter away from having lost an inch off my waist and with a month to spare. So I changed the goal to losing two inches in two months.

From now on, I accept that struggling is a part of life. No resistance here!

Someday Is Now

Do you think about "someday?" As in, "Someday, I will be thin, happy, fulfilled, in love, a supermodel, a published writer…[insert goal of your choice here]." The future "someday" has an underlying fantasy element in it. It implies that all of this will just happen automagically. There is no responsibility, and also no control, therefore anxiety. Take responsibility for today, gain control and reduce anxiety. The real "today" means doing whatever you need to get done to reach your goal.

Usually this kind of pep talk makes me roll my eyes, but it's something I actually wrote in 2005 when I was all fired up and actively losing weight. I discovered it while looking back through some old files. It's important to remember that taking small steps today, no matter what it is I want in life, makes all the difference in how I feel about myself.

Tim and I were treated to a two-hour cruise on the Connecticut River, followed by dinner at an historic restaurant. It was a second annual event and as we boarded the boat and found a spot to sit, my thoughts drifted back to the previous year's event, which led me to remember how I felt about myself then.

I'd felt desperate, unhappy, angry, and ugly…wallowing in self-pity, insecurity, and defensiveness. And no, it wasn't PMS. I noted that, sort of like the absence of noise (versus the presence of silence), those feelings were absent on this cruise. I felt peaceful, confident, content, and dare I say it – beautiful.

Does this mean I am now thin as a supermodel? Ha! No. The big difference is that I'm not worried about my perceived failures. I'm not worried about "someday." My confidence in myself has given me the ability to be open and fair, and to deal appropriately not only with others but also myself...versus being defensive, offensive, and inappropriately reactive.

A Funny Thing Happened
On The Way To Acceptance

Carrying over the "someday is now" theme, how many times have you heard "it's the journey – not the destination"? I've heard it, and thought it, and said it about 306 trillion times. And how many times have I assumed that the arc of my journey will end when I reach my destination? How often have I assumed that my journey is an arc? A lot.

I'm fascinated by the fact that it takes time, sometimes a long time, to "get" something you think you already know – to "get it" on a cellular level. I thought I was all about my journey – a total journey woman! But in the back of my mind was the idea that sooner or later I'd get to my destination – preferably sooner.

Sometimes I sense that my journey is painful (frustrating? annoying?) for others to witness, especially for those who know me well, or for those who love me. Heck, it's been painful, frustrating, and annoying for me at times! When I think back on all the things I've tried, all the machinations I've put myself through in the name of…what? Arriving at my destination after having traveled an arc-shaped journey?

The journey has NOT been an arc. An arc implies taking off, moving lightly up, up, and up, and then gently down, down and down until you land. My journey has been more like a hurtling flight, with moments of stomach-dropping turbulence, a lot of general bumpiness, and even a fair amount of smooth, effortless gliding. All the while I've kept at it, trying to stay in control of the rudder and the stabilizer.

At this juncture, the flight has been rather smooth and pleasant. I've been able to relax and enjoy the ride, only needing small adjustments to maintain my flight path.

When I decided that my journey was moving from struggle to acceptance, acceptance became my destination and I shunned struggle. Then I accepted struggle as part of the deal. Now here's the funny part: acceptance is no longer my destination. It's part of the same deal. It's my journey.

A Laborious Mosaic

"There are very few human beings who receive the truth, complete
and staggering, by instant illumination.
Most of them acquire it fragment by fragment,
on a small scale, by successive developments,
cellularly, like a laborious mosaic."
~ Anais Nin

Isn't that what I was just saying?

I attended an event at which actress/author Jamie Lee Curtis was the keynote speaker. She spoke about how important the truth is to her, and included the above quote from Anais Nin. And to illustrate why the truth is often so hard to know, and how often the truth is not pretty, she also recited a passage from the Talmud:

You don't see things as they are; you see them as you are.

She spoke about how she came to be in the place she is today – being a mom to a son with learning issues, writing children's books, doing Activia commercials, and speaking to groups of women like the one of which I was a part. She asked, "How did I get to this place?"

In answer to her own question, she recited the Serenity Prayer:

God grant me the serenity to accept the things I cannot change;
Courage to change the things I can;

And the wisdom to know the difference.

"It's all about acceptance," Jamie Lee added.

She pointed out how so many people use addiction to avoid self-acceptance: food, alcohol, technology, shopping, celebrity, plastic surgery, and so on. She noted the two extremes of obesity and anorexia nervosa, and the fact that it's hard to know what "normal" is anymore.

"What women do to themselves because they are not satisfied with what they see, with who they really are, is staggering," she said. "What they do to themselves makes it so they can't see themselves as they really are. And in the end it doesn't work because when they look at themselves in the mirror, they see the fraud, they see the lie." And so, the cycle continues.

Jamie Lee related that she felt lucky to have received the truth in an illuminating moment. On the day that Princess Diana died, Jamie Lee had turned to a book of Buddhist meditations that she'd been given.

"I am not into meditating, but I thought the book would impress my friends," she joked. "But that day, I picked it up and read the introduction and it started off like this: 'Someone who is living mindfully, at the moment of their death, asks themselves two questions: Did I live wisely? Did I love well?'"

She reminded us about the life Diana had chosen to live versus the life she was supposed to live. "She is someone who had definitely learned how to live wisely and who had loved well. And ever since then, at the end of every day, I ask myself those two questions: Did I live wisely? Did I love well? It has become the framework for my life."

For me, Jamie Lee's talk wasn't an instant illumination, but yet another fragment in the laborious mosaic that is my life.

A Q-and-A With Myself

"Many people have been taught that they can't have what they want and that a life full of struggle is somehow more honorable than one of joy.
Unlearn this lesson!
It's not selfish to seek pleasure in our thoughts, relationships, and vocation.
Life is meant to be lived joyfully!"
~ Dr. Christiane Northrup

When did I learn that I can't have what I want and that life is a struggle? And how do I unlearn this lesson?

Why is it that progress in the joy department can seemingly be undone by just a day or two of feeling hopeless and pitiful and sorry for myself?

Why does my life seem so hopeless at times?

And why do I feel like "why bother?"

And why do I feel like a failure?

Why was I given this body...a body that is extra thick in the middle and only getting thicker?

And why do I feel so hopeless as it concerns ridding my body of this extra fat especially when I've been given all the tools and knowledge I need?

And why do I feel so rotten right now?

And why do I feel like I am not living up to my potential?

And why can't I love my body EVERY day?

And why do I have to have days like this?

And why, when I know it's not a permanent feeling, does it feel like it is?

And why do I wish I were someone else?

My life is so much more wonderful than not.

So far, I have experienced a lot of success.

I have discovered my gifts and am able to use and share them with others!

I have incredible core strength and balance.

I live in a comfortable and safe home in a beautiful little city.

I have accomplished many things that I never thought possible!

I have an incredible husband who loves me so completely, unapologetically and unconditionally and even better, I love him completely, unapologetically and unconditionally.

I know that "days like this" are a part of life and that it will be okay.

I believe that everything works out the way it is supposed to.

I am so blessed to be me. This is how I practice.

Part III:
The Physical Reality

November 2009

*"What you see depends mainly
on what you look for."*
~ Sir John Lubbock

My Journey Continues,
But On A Different (Naturo)Path

I've been told that asking "why" shuts us down, while asking "how" opens up possibilities.

Instead of "why do I feel this way?" it's more helpful to ask "how can I feel the way I want to feel?" or "how can I change the way I feel about my body?"

I know this to be true, but sometimes I'm not in the mood to practice it. Sometimes I feel like wallowing. Sometimes I'm in the midst of a hormonal snit and I know it won't be long before my mood evens out and I will be open to the possibilities once again.

One of those possibilities was naturopathic medicine. A woman I know mentioned that she had been to a naturopath who had helped her address some health issues that, while not serious, were impacting her quality of life. And then my chiropractor mentioned that there's a naturopath who shares office space with him.

But, as with most things, it took me some time to be ready to take this step.

I haven't been feeling "myself" for the past few months. I've been fatigued and not sleeping well. My midsection seems to be expanding, despite some of the positive changes I've made and been consistent with. A part of me believes it was just a matter of age, shifting hormones, and the onset of perimenopause...although I have no proof. And so I was just going to say "the hell with it," and give in to whatever time had in store for me.

Another part of me said, "Hell, no, you shouldn't just accept it as a matter of fact." And then there's that part of me that blames me for things that might not really be my fault, that beats me up for not being perfect or for being unwilling to even try and be perfect.

You know how you can "know" something in your gut, but because it seems easier you choose to ignore it? I think it's called denial.

Well, denial is no longer working for me.

I went to see the naturopath and after spending 90-plus minutes going over my history and answering questions that no doctor has ever asked me, I now know a lot more about myself:

- I've been on birth control pills for 25 years and should have stopped taking them when I married 12 years ago (Tim had a vasectomy).
- My instinct regarding my thyroid levels was spot on (meaning I had a feeling that they may be "off"), even though my doctor said my TSH was "okay but borderline."
- My seasonal depression may be due to lack of vitamin D, even though I thought I was taking enough.

The naturopath was especially concerned about the birth control pills and the effect they may be having on my estrogen levels. Based on my answers to some of her questions, she believes I have too much estrogen in my body! And it bothers me that, over the past five years I have discussed stopping the birth control with my doctor and she's always had a rather blasé response: "If you're not having any problems with it, there's no need to stop taking them."

And all of this may be why it's so incredibly hard for me to lose weight. I say that even though there's a nagging little voice in the back of my mind saying, "Okay, Karen, whatever you say. We know you're just looking for another excuse...we know that the reason you aren't losing any weight is because you're not TRYING and because you're lazy and unmotivated!"

So based on the naturopath's recommendation, I quit the birth control pills and I eliminated all the supplements I'd been taking. She also recommended a homeopathic remedy and a liver support supplement that will help flush out and detox my system. In three weeks, I'll have full blood work done. She will then add in specific supplements depending on the results.

This all happened the day after my 47th birthday. I arrived at this fork in the road with frustration, but I chose a direction and I continue the journey feeling peaceful. I know there may be some discomfort ahead and that this leg of the journey might take some time, but I am looking forward to healing.

Another Stop On The (Naturo)Path

It's been three weeks since my initial visit with my naturopath and there have been changes – some major and some so minor that I didn't even realize it until she asked me specific questions.

Here's what I noticed (in no particular order):

- I'd been bleeding on and off – sometimes heavily and painfully – since quitting the Pill and I met my ovaries for the first time in 25 years. The naturopath was not concerned about any of this and said it will take some time for my body to get regulated.
- A chronic rash on my left pinky finger cleared up (this is one of those minor things I hadn't even considered until she asked).
- Fewer cravings for carbs and feeling slightly more "in control."
- Feeling more accepting in general. This is something I'd noticed on my own, but she also asked specifically if I felt better about myself and not so self-critical. I was surprised that she'd noticed.

The next step – blood work: full lipid panel (cholesterol), metabolic panel (glucose, electrolyte and fluid balance, kidney function, and liver function), complete blood count, iron, complete thyroid panel (TSH, T4, free T3, and anti TPO), vitamin B12, vitamin D, and Lyme disease. My blood draw filled seven vials!

She added fish oil to my regimen, upped the dosage of the homeopathic remedy, and recommended making it a point to eat 75 grams of protein per day. Remember when I made all those pronouncements about sugar and protein? Well, the fact is I haven't been tracking my food intake.

Once the birth control pills are out of my system, she wants me to see a hormone specialist. She thought I might be "estrogen dominant" and low on progesterone. In two weeks, we'll have a follow-up. For the first time in a long time, I don't feel like I'm spinning my wheels! I don't feel like I'm grasping at straws and looking for some magic pill.

Temporary Sanity

When I started writing this chapter, it was going to be all about how I had turned a corner, how I was no longer being ruled by sugar and that life would be perfect from now on. I wrote:

Something amazing happened yesterday. A friend invited me over for a cookie-making party. Everyone would make a batch then we'd all share so we could bring home a variety of cookies. Now, in the past, this kind of event would have resulted in a major sugar binge that would last for days. And in the back of my mind, I'd be excited and slightly desperate, although I wouldn't show it outwardly. I'd be thinking that it's Christmas and this is what happens at Christmas, except the food/drink orgy would just continue well past the holidays until I felt horrible, both mentally and physically.

None of that happened. I ate two cookies yesterday and that was it. There was no temptation. No desire. No secret desperation. I sent the batch with Tim to work today to share with his co-workers, which was my intention anyway. I don't know if it's just a passing thing? Is it the yogurt I eat every day now? The homeopathic remedy? The fact that I still have a cold? Is my body balancing out? Will I feel this way next time I'm at a party? I know I've had brief and temporary phases like this before and there's a small(er) voice in the back of my brain telling me it's just a phase and I can't possibly be healing for real. But this time it feels different. Am I healing or was it just another brief and temporary foray into food sanity?

But no. It was temporary sanity. Within 24 hours I was back in an old pattern of shifty-eyed denial knowing my husband wouldn't be home for three days. That out-of-control feeling came back and insanity ruled the day: organic cheese puffs, chocolate, a granola bar and a couple glasses of wine.

I put my halo back on and had yogurt, berries and walnuts for breakfast, kickboxed for 90 minutes, then had a healthy lunch. But instead of making myself some dinner, I ate half a loaf of white bread with butter.

It caught up with me in the morning in the form of bloat, unsettled bowels, and that empty-itchy-angry-distracted-hate-myself feeling (and the guilt that comes from knowing I'm not walking my talk, and then the underlying pain that comes from being too hard on myself)...which leads me to eat, which leads me to feel crappier, which leads me to isolate myself, and not reach out because I feel like a hypocrite.

But this time I didn't do that. I chose to reach out and my friends helped me and it made me cry. And I cried and cried. And I felt a little better. And this is a tenuous moment because I am feeling that "I've-been-a-bad-girl" feeling, which at first causes me to abstain, but then leads to self-abuse.

I'm *not* going there. I am *not* going there. I *will not* go there.

So let me go here instead: I've made some huge strides in the past year. I have become aware of things that I was not aware of a year ago. Now that I know better, I do better, most of the time. Food insanity happens, but with less frequency and less intensity. If I really think about it, I am more often sane than insane regarding food. I am taking steps, both physically and mentally, to heal myself. This is progress. It's okay. I am okay.

Feelings Are Not Facts

I had an unspoken realization. So I will speak of it now. I am still seeking a magic solution. There's a little voice in the back of my head that believes the naturopath will discover something wrong with me that, once fixed and/or healed, will make me skinny. Conversely, there's another voice in my head that says, "Face it, Karen, you're a loser and that's the reason you always fail miserably. Suck it up and suffer. Work out until you can't move and starve yourself. That's the only way this will work."

It's that "all or nothing" thinking again.

I know I am not a loser...but it feels that way sometimes. And then I remember that feelings aren't facts. I acknowledge that I slipped, fell and got back up again with lightning speed this time. And that, along with being able to understand my thought processes, is huge.

In addition, I've begun to understand that it's not about how I look, but about how I feel, both mentally and physically. Where I used to be more concerned about how I look, I am now more concerned with how I feel. And where I used to be able to binge on sugar and feel okay, I most certainly cannot now. And the sick physical feelings directly equate to sick mental feelings. My little breakdown was an opportunity, not a catastrophe.

The Voices In My Head

I've been reading about eating disorders. Many of the stories are about anorexia nervosa and binge/purge syndrome. I admit that I have preconceived ideas about eating disorders and I have often looked at photos of women who have them and thought, "She looks beautiful and healthy." But I also feel their sense of desperation, struggle, shame and hopelessness and I wonder, "Where is the disconnect?"

I have always considered anorexia nervosa and bulimia to be true disorders or mental illnesses, compared to just plain old bingeing and being obese (which for me was just a sign that I am a weak, lazy person). I grew up in a family that prizes strength, perseverance, and health and abhors weakness, laziness, people who give up, and illness of any sort. I recognize that I sometimes feel the same way.

I used the words "disordered eating" to describe my behavior in response to a question my naturopath asked me. Because I sometimes think of myself as a weak, lazy person I always look for an explanation as to why I just can't control myself: a rebellious inner child? Addiction to sugar? Some sort of physical imbalance? A chemical imbalance? And as I write this, I think, "There you go, Karen, looking to blame your problems on someone or something else." And as I write this I realize that the word "blame" implies that shame needs to be involved too. And when there is blame and shame, there is defensiveness. And defensiveness leads to denial.

Admitting a problem requires some sort of action. I've made proclamations. I've committed to plans. I've received counseling. I've taken classes. I've been inspired to create new and unique goals. I poured a bottle of wine down the drain. But have I really followed through? Yes and no. I'm eating a lot less sugar than I used to, I'm drinking a whole lot less wine than I used to, and I'm still working out faithfully. But my waist hasn't changed. And I still binge. And when I do, I still feel like a pathetic, weak, lazy loser.

I don't like the idea that there might be "something wrong with me." I've touched on this before: I grew up in a family where a lot of accusing went on, even in the name of concern. Accusations lead to denial. "There's nothing wrong with me, I choose to be this way, so just leave me alone."

I understand that many people who overcome one addiction often trade it for another. I've read about women who, in overcoming an eating disorder, turn to drinking in order to deal with it. I've read about women who, after having gastric bypass surgery, become sex addicts. I know that I sometimes go shopping in order to avoid sugar. Is it that we're all just looking to fill some emotional void or might it actually be physiological? I've always hated the word "addiction" because I associate it with an accusation. But I'll use it anyway.

People don't like being sick or addicted. People don't do it on purpose. It doesn't feel good to say, "but I can't help it" even when I *can't* seem to help it. The idea of being able to talk myself out of it appeals to me, but after 40-plus years of trying, I get that it doesn't work. The idea of a 12-step group does not appeal to me, although I know it works for many. Other support groups, both in real life and online, have been wonderful for me and I will continue to seek them out.

Might I have an undiagnosed mental illness? The more I think about it, the more I believe that mental illness is just a big continuum and we're all on it. The stigmas and myths associated with mental illness are being broken down. This is by no means a self-diagnosis, but the more I understand about addiction and eating disorders, the more I understand what the hell I've been struggling with

And the voices in my head say:

"She just doesn't get it. All she has to do is eat less and exercise more."

"She did it once before and lost 50+ pounds, why can't she do it now? She must not want it badly enough."

"Okay, she wants to call it an eating disorder or a mental illness now. Whatever."

"She's always scheming for an easy answer."

It's enough to make me crazy.

It's Not In My Head – It's In My Blood

My naturopath got the results of my blood work and her instincts proved accurate – but the results also brought a few surprises. She said that I have Lyme disease and a "sluggish" thyroid, as well as Epstein-Barr virus, low vitamin D, and low vitamin B12. Otherwise, I am fine.

I don't think I realized just how nervous I'd been about this. I'd felt rather "low" and full of dread prior to the appointment, which I'd chalked up to hormones. But I think I was also anxious about getting the results. When she told me about the Lyme disease, I burst into tears...relieved in some ways, and scared in others.

In the scheme of things, it's not a big deal, but it sort of presented a shift in what I thought my reality was. I think the symptoms (stiff/achy joints, fatigue, low energy, difficulty taking off weight, depression) came on slowly over time and I attributed them to age, weight, and working out. I'd gotten used to feeling this way and so I didn't complain too much – which was influenced by my upbringing. The idea that some or all of these symptoms might go away thrills me.

The Lyme needed treating first. My doctor says she's treated hundreds of patients with Lyme using a homeopathic remedy – a series of ten treatments taken every three days for a month, along with an immune system booster. I'd rather treat it this way than with the megadoses of antibiotics typically prescribed (and which don't always work).

After the Lyme treatment, she'll treat the Epstein-Barr and we'll look at my hormones and adrenal function (which are tested via saliva). She also gave me vitamin D to take by itself, which will help with depressed feelings and help boost my immunity. I am excited to move forward and to feel better and while I acknowledge that it will take time, it's going to take longer than I want it to.

The Gift Of Knowledge And Acknowledgement

After Christmas, many of my friends and family talked about their favorite gifts. It didn't take me long to realize that the best gift I could have ever given myself was that initial appointment with the naturopath.

I have to admit that I am still in shock regarding everything I am facing, health-wise. It challenges assumptions (both positive and negative) that I had made about myself and it took some time to adjust what I now consider a new reality. Then I became excited about the possibilities.

I do not have cancer or AIDS. There's no death sentence. But these issues have definitely affected my quality of life both physically and mentally. It feels really good to know that I know I don't have to suck it up any more. "It" being the symptoms I just assumed were due to age, weight gain (which in and of itself is a symptom), and, if I am honest, some sort of character flaw.

I've decided to keep my focus on myself and not what anyone else says. I am going with the premise that as I move forward with the various treatments, I will feel better.

I am looking forward to:

- sleeping better
- having more energy

- not having waves of fatigue wash over me at random time during the day
- running again without feeling like I am going to break
- kickboxing without feeling like I've been beaten up afterwards
- recovering my enthusiasm for running and kickboxing!
- sharpening of my mental focus
- reducing the "haze" I sometimes feel in my brain
- waking up feeling refreshed
- waking up (or standing up after having been sitting for a while) without my joints screaming
- muscles that don't feel tired/achy/rusty for no good reason
- not feeling depressed, weak, lazy, or "less than" because of these symptoms

Yes, this is what I've been putting up with and "accepting" for I don't know how long. There are times when these symptoms seem to worsen, and times when they're not so bad. But now that I know they aren't my fault, why I have them, and that they will go away...I readily acknowledge them.

ϡ

The Truth Sets Me Free,
Or Something Like That

Here's the uncomfortable truth: I lied to my mother about having Lyme disease because I didn't want to deal with her reaction. I allowed myself to believe it was a matter of self-protection, but then wondered why I felt so awful. I also realized that my defensiveness was sending a message: "I don't trust myself."

I am learning to exercise a weak muscle...

...the it's-okay-if-my-mother-is-angry-with-me muscle

...the it's-okay-if-my-mother-thinks-I-am-stupid muscle

...the oh-I've-created-a-prison-for-myself-but-now-it's-time-to-set-myself-free muscle.

For too long I've censored myself around my mother, especially where certain topics are concerned, because I don't want conflict over how I live my life and the decisions I make. And if I am honest, I see that censoring myself has not only led me to lie, it's led me to become inauthentic.

So, I chose to be honest with her.

In an email, I wrote, in part:

"The truth is that I do have Lyme disease and didn't want to tell you until after I had been treated.... The truth is that I didn't want to deal

with your reaction to my news.... I am uncomfortable that I lied to you. I own that.

...I have been censoring myself around you concerning certain subjects because I don't want conflict over how I live my life and the decisions I make. You and I are two very different people and we handle our lives in different ways – not right or wrong, just different.

I think boundaries are a good and healthy thing for the both of us, so from now on I will be honest and tell you when I don't want to talk about a certain subject and I hope that you will respect my wish and trust that I'll do the right thing. I like being open and honest, even if you don't agree with me, or approve of how I am handling certain aspects of my life."

I've been thinking about my role in the bigger picture – that I let myself and my mother down because I didn't create a healthy boundary. And that led me to be angry and defensive.

In my quest to have a good relationship, I thought that all I needed to do was be loving and supportive, but without the appropriate boundary, I became fake and inauthentic instead. I was all nicey-nice. I made such a point of avoiding conflict with my mother, that in the end, conflict was all I felt when I was around her or spoke to her.

That's *my* issue.

Health Issues?? Moi?

I was discussing with some friends my Lyme disease and other diagnoses, and I told them how, many months ago before I knew better, I'd started feeling sorry for myself – guilty, stupid, whiny, and all those other useless I'm-a-loser-beat-myself-up emotions.

I told them it was hard for me to be consistent with my workouts because my joints hurt. My body hurt. I was tired. And I was getting depressed. Vicious cycle stuff.

I told them how I yearned for the day when I would feel like my old self, like the powerhouse I used to be.

And then I got a sign – my knees stopped hurting. I described it as being like the absence of noise. You know when there's some low-level monotonous noise in the background for a long time and then all of a sudden it's gone and you think, "Oh, I didn't realize that noise was making so much noise!" And then you feel relief. That's what I am feeling right now. Does that mean the Lyme treatment is working?!

Anyway, one of my friends said that she was sorry to hear about my recent health issues.

Whoa. Stop right there. HEALTH ISSUES?? Who me? I don't have health issues. I am fine.

That's exactly what went through my mind when she said "health issues." And then I immediately realized where that thought came from: the old family programming that being sick is somehow a personality flaw and that the tick who bit me and gave me Lyme disease must have known that I wasn't eating right and exercising, because that's the root of all evil right there.

What Is Your Intention When You Eat?

I'm starting to believe that the intention with which we eat something matters most. Eating out of guilt, rebellion, desperation, or any other so-called "negative" emotion will almost always have a negative impact. You might argue that eating joyfully can also have a negative impact, and that's true, but when I really examine why I am eating and what I am eating as a result, then joyful eating is never bad.

That came to me while reading others' accounts of sneaking food.

I am a food sneaker from way back and I think I did it out of rebellion. Like many children, I was sometimes forced to eat foods I hated, even if it meant eating them cold for breakfast the next day, or eating what I had tried to swallow and gagged up. To this day, I can't eat foods with a certain texture: lima beans, peas, kidney beans, black beans, pretty much beans of any kind, mashed potatoes or liver...blech. I don't blame my parents because I honestly don't think they knew any better, besides there were starving children in China and they didn't want me to be spoiled or ungrateful.

Then when I was a little older, my mother might raise an eyebrow or make a comment if I wanted more of something than she thought I should have. So to get back at them, I'd sneak foods I liked: cookies and crackers mostly. I'd look forward to being left home alone, or to being given a babysitting or pet sitting job. I loved to raid other people's cabinets and see what kinds of goodies they had. Of course, I'd try and hide the evidence. It's when the bingeing started. Now I can look back at that girl with a sense of compassion rather than harsh judgment. When I think about that now, and from the perspective of my own adult self, I know I wasn't fooling anyone.

Even just a year ago that wouldn't have been possible.

Another thing I realize is that I don't have to sneak food any more because no one is judging me and so I can truly enjoy my food.

I say this as much for myself as for anyone who is reading this: slow down, relax, be grateful for your food, and eat it joyfully and with pleasure. Take the time to taste and savor it. Think about why you're eating and the underlying feelings that accompany the act of eating.

Why Am I Resentful
When I Should Be Grateful?

For some reason wine no longer agrees with me. If I have a glass, I wake up in the middle of the night sweating, uneasy, queasy, and heart pounding. Next to someone ELSE being nauseated, my biggest fear is being nauseated myself! I'm talking heart-pounding panic attacks.

This happened on three separate occasions in two months. The only things I can connect this reaction to are the treatments for Lyme disease and Epstein-Barr virus. Or maybe it's hormonal.

The only other time I've had this reaction to wine was when flying. The first time it happened (I'd had one glass), I thought it was just a fluke. When it happened a second time (two glasses), I decided I'd never drink on a plane again.

Now, I've also struggled with what I call my "wine habit." What bothered me most were the empty calories because more often than not, it was the glass(es) of wine that would be put me over "the limit" on calories, not to mention making me hungrier and less apt to care about mindless snacking in the evening.

But now here I am, scared to drink wine. You'd think I'd be grateful but I am, in fact, resentful. Something that I used to enjoy has been made scary and unpleasant. On an intellectual level I know it's better for me that I don't drink wine, but I feel like a child whose favorite toy has been taken away. It's not fair.

I Am Finally In My Right Brain

I spent most of my life finding it difficult to do much of anything without first asking my friends, my mother, my husband, for advice. I didn't trust myself to make decisions and was in constant need of input, approval and reassurance.

Then one day I made a choice that changed my life – a choice that freed me to just go ahead and do things without needing advice and approval and allowed me to see myself in a whole new way.

I spent many years as a writer/reporter for various plastics industry trade publications, mostly for publishing companies and trade associations. I enjoyed this work because I was able to travel extensively throughout the United States and Europe. It was rather glamorous and at a time when air travel was far more civilized than it is today.

I also liked it because when someone asked what I did for a living, I could reply, "I am a writer." You see, I'd wanted to be a writer since I was in seventh grade. And when I went to college, I went with the intention of becoming a writer. I didn't have specific plans, although the idea of being a foreign correspondent was attractive. I imagined that I'd start at a newspaper. I also thought I might write a novel. Or a children's book.

But here's what happened instead. A friend who'd graduated a semester early got a job at a public relations agency in New York City. She told me they had plenty of openings for assistant-type jobs and that it was a great way to break into PR. So off I went, with no clue and no plan. I hated PR. After a year or so I left and got a job as an editorial assistant at a small magazine publishing company that served the model airplane market. Again, I had no real plan or goal, I wanted to write.

About a year later, I discovered plastics. I went to work for a magazine published by a plastics industry trade association and spent 17 years at various magazines, eventually becoming Editor-In-Chief of one publication.

And then it was over. The magazine was sold to a large corporation in California and the new owners didn't want me. I cast about thinking that one of the other magazines might hire me, or at least use me as a contributor on a freelance basis. I even offered my services to local plastics processors and equipment manufacturers. Those efforts went nowhere.

In hindsight, I know that I had absolutely no confidence in myself in those 17 years as a reporter, writer or editor. And I think everyone sensed it. And so I told myself that I'd never write again. That was in 2003.

I went to work for a local Borders bookstore that opened in August of 2003. After six months as a bookseller, I was asked to become the Corporate Sales representative and did very well, considering that "sales" was something I thought I hated! That position put me out in the community, attending networking events and meeting everyone from small business owners to executives and managers at larger companies. I found myself talking more about my previous career than my current one, and often, I was encouraged to start freelancing.

So I quit the Corporate Sales representative position, started working part time in the stock room, and focused on freelancing. I joined the local Chamber of Commerce (which resulted in a lot of business-to-business work) and pitched a story idea to the editor of *Grace* magazine. The editor wasn't interested in the idea I had at the time but said she had another story and would I take it? I jumped at it of course, but at the same time said to myself, "Are you crazy?" In the back of my mind I thought, "I didn't know how to write about anything other than plastics, and even that I didn't do well."

The assignment was simple: write about how getting clothes altered to fit well makes all the difference in how you feel about yourself. I did the interviews and research and wrote the article.

And here's that all-important life-changing decision: I didn't ask any of my friends or family to read the article before I submitted it.

This was a conscious, premeditated decision. When I hit "send" on the email to submit the article I felt both scared to death AND triumphant! Somehow I knew, deep down inside, that it was time for me to trust that I'd done a good job and that I didn't need anyone else's approval or reassurance.

The results of this one moment have been unfolding ever since. It's not like I went from being one way (needing constant reassurance and approval) to being the opposite (100% confident all the time). There are times when I can't believe that people think I am talented or that I have something valuable to offer.

I thought about my college aspirations of being a journalist and how it never quite worked out the way I thought it would. And then I took one of those silly quizzes on Facebook ("Are You Right-Brained or Left-Brained?") and saw that one of the questions lumped "journalist" in with such left-brained occupations as engineer, doctor, and accountant. I spent all those years trying to force myself into a more left-brained kind of career because it involved writing.

As it turns out, I am most definitely right-brained. After I posted the results, the comments that followed were along the lines of: "You needed to take this test?" and "Well, duh!" I responded that while it may come as a surprise, I hadn't realized this about myself until recently. And until that moment, I don't think I had given myself permission to embrace this about myself. I knew it, but I didn't KNOW it.

Before, I didn't believe that I was a writer because I wasn't doing the kind of writing that suits me or plays to my strengths. Now I am truly a writer. That's who I am at my core.

So what does all of this have to do with weight? Writing on my terms and being confident in myself fills up that empty place that I have often turned to food to fill. I can see how my confidence in myself as a writer mirrors my confidence in my body and vice versa. At one time I thought that weight loss was the key to all happiness and confidence but when I began writing for myself, I could see that it wasn't. Writing for myself helps me to better love myself and that translates to making better choices for my health.

A Quick Health Update

So I finally went to see the hormone specialist and it was at once wonderful and terrifying. He pretty much confirmed – as much as he could without the results of blood work and saliva tests – that I am estrogen dominant, that my progesterone is probably too low, that my thyroid is just enough out of whack to be causing certain symptoms, and that my cortisol levels are also probably out of whack.

Developing heart disease worries me, as it runs on both sides of my family, and I know I already have a couple of risk factors. The good news is that I have some really good habits that counter-act heart disease, but I can do more! All of this can and will be addressed.

However, some of the old (family) tapes have been playing in my head and that's why it's terrifying for me. Illness of any sort was never dealt with in a healthy way (pun not intended) and so I don't know how to be anything other than scared or guilty. But I am learning and I am letting go.

Dealing with it "in a healthy way" involves saliva tests, taking my temperature first thing in the morning (a lower than normal temperature on waking can indicate a thyroid issue), and getting another round of blood work done. The blood work will show my real risk for heart disease, along with some other things. Filling out the symptom checklist for the saliva test, I kept coming across things that made me think, "Oh...so that's why I feel this way." It's likely I'll be prescribed a bioidentical progesterone cream that has a slew of benefits, including lowering blood pressure and cholesterol, and acting as a natural anti-depressant and anti-anxiety agent. And, Lord knows, my anxiety can go through the roof.

Did I Speak Too Soon?

I feel like I've regressed, health-wise. My joints hurt, my muscles ache, and I have days when I am oh-so-tired, even though I am getting plenty of sleep.

Did the Lyme treatment fail? Or do the aches have to do with ridding my body of Epstein-Barr (EB) virus? Or is it due to the potential thyroid/hormone/adrenal issues?

I know that chronic Lyme causes symptoms that mimic chronic fatigue syndrome, fibromyalgia, "brain fog," and depression. I know that people who have chronic Lyme do not always respond to the traditional two-to-four-week antibiotic treatment. I know that many doctors do not/will not "recognize" that chronic Lyme exists and the traditional tests used to detect Lyme are often "false negative" *especially* in people who have had Lyme for a long time. I know that there are doctors – referred to as Lyme-Literate MDs or LLMDs – who do recognize chronic Lyme and who recommend long stints (like up to a year) of antibiotic treatment.

Maybe I am not cured. So what do I do now?

A part of me doesn't believe I had/have Lyme because it wasn't diagnosed "traditionally." Do I trust what my naturopath says or do I go elsewhere and get more tests and try other treatment? Should I consult my regular doctor or see a LLMD?

After talking or corresponding with several people I know who have dealt with Lyme in various ways, I sat quietly and thought things over. I decided not to worry about it and finish out my EB treatment. I will address any thyroid/hormone/ adrenal issues once the results of saliva and other blood work are in. And in a month I will ask my naturopath to order me another Lyme test. If there's an improvement and my numbers are in the "okay" range, I will trust that the homeopathic remedy worked. I will continue to monitor how I feel and maybe do another round of the remedy. If my numbers have not improved, I will make an appointment with a LLMD and consider long-term antibiotic treatment.

In the meantime the lesson has been driven home once again: the key to everything is acceptance of what is. And it takes constant practice.

It's All Good, But I Need To Vent

I've been so emotional. And scattered. And unable to focus. I had a little meltdown at kickboxing and started crying right in the middle of doing crunches because my neck hurt. Then my contact lens came out and I went to the bathroom and cried some more. Came back and finished class then cried some more when everyone asked what was wrong...all I could say is "my body hurts and I'm hormonal." I wasn't crying from the pain...it's not THAT bad.

I think I'm feeling that it's all over for me. Not that I have some life-threatening illness, but that my quality-of-life is being threatened. I spent most of my 20s and 30s fat, inactive, and insecure, and then I lost all this weight, got active, got excited, loved pushing myself, and then BAM it's over. My 15 minutes is up.

I feel like I've opened the proverbial can of worms, or maybe it's Pandora's Box.

The more I look into all these issues, the more issues keep popping up. I'm tired of dealing with it and am tempted to close the lid again. And if I do, am I closing the lid on the one element that will make all the difference?

Ever since I started this process with the naturopath, all I've gotten is bad news. I feel worse than when I started. Yeah, my energy was lagging a bit and I had some aches and pains, but I was thinking there'd be some gentle answer, like "here, take some herbs and you'll feel better." But no. What I got was Lyme disease and Epstein Barr and hormonal hell.

My rational, positive side understands that the treatments will make me feel worse before I feel better and that going off birth control pills threw my body into a tizzy. I now see that birth control pills masked a lot of things.

The results of my blood and saliva tests came back; I am excited and scared at the same time. Mostly, I just want to feel better. I want to feel vibrant and like myself. I don't want any more bad news or treatments that make me feel like crap.

Oh, and on top of all of this? I feel guilty because I have friends who ARE dealing with life-threatening illnesses and who are receiving treatments that make what I am going through look like a walk in the park.

On a side note, for the first time...ever? I don't care what I look like or how much I weigh. All I care about is how I feel physically. When I think about all the anguish I had over the number on the scale it seems rather silly. So, yeah, I'm feeling a little sorry for myself...I am a little uncomfortable physically. But you know what else? My life rocks. It's all good.

I Want To Thank My Body

At my first appointment with the hormone specialist, I was terrified because I thought the results of my blood work would indicate serious issues like heart disease or being pre-diabetic. I'd already been on Lipitor for more than ten years and I get my cholesterol and glucose checked every year. The numbers have always been good. But the hormone specialist wanted to look at other risk factors for cardiovascular disease...like C-reactive protein (which indicates inflammation) and the size and quality of HDL/LDL particles. Were these more worms to let out of the can? More escapees from Pandora's Box?

After the follow-up appointment, I was no longer terrified.

About ten years ago, my C-reactive protein test put me in the "high risk" category for heart disease. This was well before I started losing weight and exercising. The most recent test showed my "relative cardiovascular risk" is average (based on a whole bunch of things, but specifically C-reactive protein, cholesterol, glucose, and A1C, which is the test used to determine diabetes). I am "normal." I was also pleased to find out that my HDL and LDL particles are "large and buoyant" versus "small and dense," which is a good thing.

There was one number that the doctor didn't like: my Coenzyme Q10 levels were on the low side of normal. I had been taking CoQ10 but the naturopath suggested not taking it while being treating for Lyme. And here's the kicker: CoQ10 helps reduce muscle and joint aches and pain, while statins (like Lipitor) can increase muscle and joint aches and pains.

Now all along I knew one of the goals of this whole deal was to stop taking Lipitor. Because my overall cardiovascular health is good (especially aspects that are not helped or affected by Lipitor), I don't need to be as concerned about my cholesterol numbers. So I am going back on CoQ10, will stop taking Lipitor, and will instead take a nutritional supplement that is designed to "Support for Healthy Blood Lipid Levels."

On the hormone front, my estrogen was normal (for a premenopausal woman), my progesterone was at the very low end of normal, but more importantly, the ratio between the two was out of range (meaning estrogen dominance, which was assumed). To help get me back in balance, he prescribed the bioidentical progesterone cream he'd suspected I would need.

I also learned about something called pregnenolone, "the mother of all hormones," and mine is on the low side of normal.

As for my cortisol (we all know it better as the belly fat producer), it's not following a "normal circadian rhythm." It's low in the morning and high at night and, according to the report, this suggests "poor blood sugar regulation and/or acute stressors that raise cortisol levels." The most common adrenal stressors that can raise cortisol levels include psychological stressors, low blood sugar, pain or injury, exposure to toxic chemicals, and infections (virus, bacteria, fungi). And I have a few of those going on, right?

So to address the cortisol and pregnenolone issues, I will be taking an adrenal calming supplement and some bioidentical pregnenolone, which will increase my levels of progesterone, as well as DHEA, a hormone produced by the adrenal glands and then converted as needed into other hormones.

He "mapped" my thyroid numbers using half circles with arrows. My numbers are all on the low side of normal and the arrows do not point in the same direction. He said the goal is the get the numbers closer to normal and have the arrows point in the same direction. He said this indicates that my thyroid is laboring (along with my adrenal glands) but there's no need for specific medication or supplements. He believes that as everything else comes into balance, my thyroid will too.

He also suggested increasing my vitamin D and fish oil intake.

Now obviously, it's going to take some time for all this to start working but I feel much more positive that these steps will help me feel better and not worse.

He wants to see me lose some more weight and I, of course, would like to do that too. Before I make any drastic changes to my diet, I want to see how I feel and what happens over the course of the next three months.

And, yeah, there's a little voice inside that thinks some weight will magically fall off and maybe it will. But that doesn't mean I'm going to revert to old, destructive habits. I've learned that lesson and I am eternally grateful to my body for taking care of me even though I used to treat it poorly.

An Ah-Ha Moment For The Record Books

"Letting go doesn't mean giving up, but rather accepting that there are things that cannot be."

"It takes more strength to let go than it does to hold on."

You know how there are "ah-ha" moments that just come to you, and there are others that have been coming for years but for some reason you just weren't ready to get it?

My latest "ah-ha" falls squarely into the latter category. I just wasn't ready. Seriously not ready.

But in 24 hours, I let something go that has weighed me down (both literally and figuratively) for more than 40 years.

I've wanted to let it go for a long time. I've turned myself inside out trying to figure out how to let it go. My husband and friends have been patient with me, supportive of me, have listened to me go on and on about this, and given me excellent advice about how to handle it. I've gotten lots of therapy too. And what's interesting is that I thought I HAD let it go, at least for a while. But I took it back because NOT letting go continued to serve me.

I knew that letting go required acceptance and I worked on it, but even though I understood it, I still couldn't/wouldn't/didn't DO it.

And I'll just say it now…I may be revisiting "it" again, but now that I have this awareness and know what it feels like, I'll be better equipped next time.

I hadn't spoken to my mother in three months. I had sent that email (in which I told her about the Lyme diagnosis and, more importantly, told her the truth about why I hadn't told her sooner), but had heard nothing in response.

A family issue unrelated to this situation prompted her to call me. I won't get into all the back and forth, but I will give myself credit for keeping my boundaries in place and for being honest.

Eventually, she brought up the issue between us and I explained (using "I" statements like a good boundary-setter) that I had felt unsupported and disrespected. She responded with "well, that's your problem" and "I'm sorry you feel that way" and "those are your feelings."

I suggested that perhaps I might come for a visit specifically so that she and I might have a couple of joint counseling sessions with her therapist. She seemed open to the idea. I told her that if I visited, I'd be more comfortable staying in a hotel and the response was "don't be ridiculous" and "you will most certainly stay here" and I said, "no, please respect and support how I feel" and I basically got a big old pfffhhhhtttt and an eye roll (yes, I could hear it over the phone).

In that moment, part of me wanted to scream at my mother. Another part of me wanted the counseling with my mother to fix everything. Another part of me never wanted to talk to her again. And yet another part of me thought, "This will just go on like it has, forever, and I will have to manage it as best I can."

And when I got off the phone, I had this exact thought: "My mother, for the most part, dismisses my feelings, interests, and thoughts, as not valid, real, or worthy, and it's been like this since I can remember."

I wasn't sad or angry. I felt free and light.

And as I processed it a little more, I changed it to: "When I talk with my mother, I feel that my feelings, interests, and thoughts are dismissed as not valid, real, or worthy."

And so my mother IS RIGHT! They *are* my feelings! And Ta-DAAA! I have the power to change them!! We've all heard it before: you can't change anyone else, all you can do is change how you feel/react in response. Just because someone says something doesn't mean it's true. How many freaking times have I said that to others??

I expect some of you reading this are thinking, "Duhhhhh." And, in fact, if I had been reading someone else's version of this same story, I might be thinking it too. It's just taken me a little longer to see it.

And here comes the hard part: acknowledging "out loud" why I needed to hang on to this for so long. I needed to be *right* about my mother and I needed others to *tell me* that I was right. In fact, that's why I wanted to see her counselor. I wanted the counselor to tell her that I am right.

It All Happens For A Reason

More and more I see that the decisions and choices we make lead us down a path...not just any old path but the path we NEED to be on. It's sort of like self-determination and fate teaming up to throw our lives in our faces. And when you start looking back at some of the seemingly insignificant decisions and choices you've made, it starts to become obvious (at least to people like me, who like to think about stuff like this) that it wasn't just me making the choice and it wasn't just fate blowing me in the wind.

I had the great fortune to attend two powerful yet unrelated events. The first was a presentation of *In Our Right Minds* by Dale Allen. It's a one-woman show billed as: "A Celebration of Women, the Sacred Feminine and the Right Brain...Guiding Women to their Strength as Leaders and Leading Men to Strength without Armor."

It blew me away with new awareness and struck harder on a chord of awareness that I've had all along...all at the same time. I took away a lot from Dale's performance.

Like this: when women shy away from, or avoid doing for themselves, they're shying away from, or avoiding doing for others. When you "do" for yourself, you "do" for others.

And this: When you model reaching your goals, achievement and success, you empower everyone around you to do the same for themselves.

But perhaps this biggest lesson for me came from listening Dale tell the story of how she came to write and produce her play in the first place.

Early one morning, after a big party in a shoreline town, she walked through the wet grass in her bare feet and sat down on a dock. She described feeling like she was 11 years old. And it came to her that she wanted to write a play, and just like any 11-year-old would, she went ahead and did it because 11-year-olds do what they want, right? There's no voice that tells them not to, that it would be stupid, or that it would be a miserable failure. When we're 11, if we want to draw a picture, we draw one! If we want to sing a song, we sing it! If we want to turn cartwheels, we turn them!

Once the play was written, she contacted a local theater about performing it. Everything started to come together. And when opening night was just a week or so away a Voice inside her head said, "STOP! Who do you think you are? You can't do this! You will fail! It will be horrible!"

She said that she understood that the Voice was trying to protect her. But at the same time she realized that the Voice didn't understand how important putting on this play was to her. And so she began to think of that Voice as a little child who needed constant reassurance. She took the Voice by the hand and coaxed it along, telling it that they could do this together. They took little steps together, took deep breaths together, and the play went on! And when the Voice realized that Dale hadn't failed or been killed outright, it was able to relax a little and Dale was able to continue on doing her thing...until she decided to take it to the next level. And the Voice came back! "STOP!!" And Dale explained that she had to do it all over again. It was a little easier the next time because the Voice trusted Dale more than it did the first time. But it was still difficult. And Dale said that each and every time she decides to take things to the next level, the Voice is there.

And here's the thing: no matter what you think you see on the outside of anyone else's successes or achievements, inside is that Voice. Everyone has it. No one is immune.

I'm starting to see that a big difference between success and failure is being able to take care of that Voice. Not "conquering" it, or even "silencing" it. You just need to take care of it, nurture it and make sure that it feels safe.

And that leads me to the second powerful event: Fitbloggin '10.

This book started out as a blog and in the time that I have been writing it, I have found a whole community of health/wellness/weight loss/fitness bloggers. It's a strong, vibrant and supportive community. Fitbloggin '10 was designed to bring us together in real life.

Now I knew long before seeing Dale's performance that there'd be plenty of opportunity for the Voice to make its appearance before, during and after Fitbloggin. And so I really had to nurture it (and I still am!). My Voice reminded me that I still haven't lost the weight I regained, that I wouldn't be able to run the 5K, that I am not as fit as some of the other attendees, that my blog isn't as popular as other blogs, blah blah blah…

And so I came up with two oaths:

> *"I will not compare myself in any regard to*

and
                          other Fitbloggin attendees"

"Supporting other Fitbloggin attendees does not require denigrating myself or downplaying my achievements!"

I even raised my right hand and swore to uphold these oaths to myself.

And then there was that moment when I spoke with a literary agent who presented at Fitbloggin about going from blog to book. She said that agents and publishers look for blogs that have at least 100,000 hits per month. So far, I get about 50,000 hits per year. The Voice was screaming at that point. But as I walked away, I told it to calm down and get used to the idea because I am still going for it! And you're now holding my dream in your hands!

One last thing I want to say about my life right this minute: I have a lot of peace in my heart – reinforced by that major "ah-ha" moment, Dale's performance, and my experience at Fitbloggin.

The peace expressed itself as what I consider to be a completely natural and healthy relationship with food while traveling. I ate what I wanted to eat, didn't obsess, didn't eat too much of anything, just enjoyed some really delicious, nourishing food in moderation. I didn't stuff myself or starve myself.

I wasn't completely oblivious because I did notice how I felt. I wondered if it might have been because I was at a conference with people who blog about diet/weight loss/health, but when I really examined it, I saw that it wasn't that. I felt filled up with other things. In the past, I would have "eaten healthy" in front of others but brought back "comfort" food to my room. I was aware that I could have done that if I wanted to, but there was no compulsion to do so.

Significant for sure.

What If I Get Stuck Like This?

Remember when I wrote about why putting on a happy face isn't always the best thing to do? I wrote: "denying negative emotions is a form of self-abuse. It's silly to put a smile on your face when what you really need to do is acknowledge feelings you might view as ugly."

So I will.

I feel heartbroken. I feel overwhelmed. I feel blank. I feel empty. I feel lonely. I feel needy. I feel like I don't care about anything. I feel uninspired. I feel let down. I feel shut down. I feel grouchy and sad. I feel unlovable.

I feel dread. What if I get stuck like this? Remember when your mother told you not to cross your eyes because they might get stuck that way? What if I get stuck?

And why do I feel this way? Is it because I only had one cup of coffee when lately I've been having two? Is it bad that I have two? It is because I'm bloated and I shouldn't be? It's not that time of the freaking month, damn it! Is it because I "feel fat"? Is it because I ate some crackers yesterday? "More than I should have?" Even though I was hungry? Is it because I thought that would never happen again, even though I knew better than to ever say that?

Yeah, I guess this is where I acknowledge that these feelings still exist inside of me. Loving myself when I feel unlovable is definitely harder than when I feel worthy.

I Am Not Stuck

I figured out why I felt:

heart broken overwhelmed underwhelmed blank empty lonely needy don't care uninspired letdown shutdown grouchy sad unlovable

It's because I had started to go down the "something is inherently wrong with me" road.

It never fails...the minute I start feeling that I need to be fixed is when I start looking outside myself for a "fix."

Filling My Heart, Not My Stomach:
A Mindstyle Change

I've been feeling rather fantastic (physically and emotionally) and I know myself well enough to know that it's partially because I'm in the "rather fantastic" part of my hormonal cycle. Without the birth control pills controlling my body, I've been able to identify a clear pattern: about two weeks of fatigue, aches, pains, anxiety, and brain fog, and about two weeks of energy, clarity, peace, and not as much pain. It remains to be seen whether Lyme disease is playing a part in all of this.

But there's something else – something beyond this current but temporary blip in the road to health.

It's a mindstyle change...like a lifestyle change but for the mind. In many ways, big and small, I've changed my mind about a lot of things that were weighing me down. I've exposed myself to new people, new thoughts, new ways of being. I've tweaked the way I think about myself, my family, friends and other aspects of my life. I've had opportunities to reach out, reach in, reach over, reach under...and I've been taking advantage of them.

I've filled my heart and mind with so much awareness and love that many of the behaviors I tend to fall back on to distract me from "what is" seem to have taken a back seat. None of this is brand new to me. It's something I've been experimenting with and practicing consistently. It's something that I knew needed to be done. It's something I know I have to continue to do.

This isn't about being perfect in either lifestyle or mindstyle. It's not about saying, "I'll never eat cheese and crackers again" or "I'll never be pissed off at my mother again." It doesn't require making huge sweeping changes all at once. It suggests being open, accepting, forgiving, and willing. It suggests understanding that I may not always feel like being open, accepting, forgiving, and willing.

I looked back at something I'd written in the past and I came across this tidbit:

"…now that I have the self-acceptance thing going, I have found myself much more willing to do the things I know are good for my body. My eyes are opened and I find myself embracing what used to seem like drudgery: counting calories, making sure I eat enough protein and fiber, avoiding "white" foods. These are all the things that support healthy weight loss, but for some reason, I had been unwilling to do them consistently. Could it be that my lack of self-acceptance made me unwilling?

Earlier this year, in one of my darker moments, I wrote "I am on a quest for the sweet spot – that balance between a healthy body weight (and image) and self acceptance right now." Add to that the idea that if I view this ("this" being that quest) as a struggle…as a fight to be fought, then that's exactly what I'll get.

It's been slow going but I think I have finally hit that sweet spot. First came self-acceptance, even though my body is still heavier than I would like it to be. From that came a real desire to discover what drives the carb cravings and "false hunger" that seem to derail me every time, that create that "struggle" and make me feel like a failure."

What I see in those words is not self-acceptance but a desperate attempt to feel it *in order to lose weight.* It wasn't an attempt to just feel good about myself. In those words I see a woman who was trying hard to feel something she doesn't in order to follow rules that lead her back to feeling unacceptable. What do you see?

A Double Whammy, Part I

For as long as I can remember, I've been told that I am "sensitive." Sometimes it's said in a positive way ("You're such a sensitive soul…") but I've also heard it accompanied with eye-rolls ("Geez! You're so sensitive!").

Along with that is another trait that has both positive and negative qualities: the ability to want to see both sides of an issue…you'll note that I don't claim to truly understand all angles of all sides – it's more of a desire to understand and to find common ground. This often gets me into trouble because I can't seem to figure out what side of an issue I am really on. And when it comes to the big issues, it hurts me (sometimes physically) when I feel conflict between people, groups, even countries. Watching the news (which I rarely do) often makes me cry.

A good example is how polarized our country has become. The hatred and anger that spews forth from both sides hurts me. It especially hurts when people close to me (family and friends) fight/argue/debate. For some reason I can't separate myself from it. I feel torn apart. And I find myself wanting to find the exact right thing to say to squelch the back and forth. Usually I do some research and find something to back up what I am trying to say. Inevitably, it comes back to bite me in the bum and I feel beaten up.

So over time I have learned to stay out of such conversations. Most of the time. But not recently. I got myself involved in several back and forth political conversations.

In the end, I was upset in ways I am still trying to figure out. The others involved probably have no clue how upset I am and I am sure the conversations have long been forgotten, but here I am still raw enough to cry over the whole thing.

Instead of trying to figure it out, I spent the last few days stuffing my face...not as severely as I might have in the past, but the desire to put handfuls of crunchy snacks into my mouth was fully engaged. I wasn't willing to fully face the bad feelings. And so I stuffed them down with Popchips, pretzel crisps, and hummus.

What's behind it (I think) is the fear that they will think I am dumb and/or that they won't like me. I am not a facts and figures kind of girl. I go with my gut much of the time.

Usually my intention is to smooth things over, but if I am honest, I will also acknowledge that there is an element of wanting, not to prove someone wrong necessarily, but to show them that their anger is misplaced or that the "facts" they cite aren't complete. To be honest, I've really come to believe that we don't/can't know the real truth about much of anything any more due to Big Media's powerful spin. And as I said, it hurts me to see people drinking from the Big Media fire hose and then turning it on others.

All of this has me questioning how I communicate, what I say, how I say it, and why I say it. It has me thinking about the example I want to set...you know, "be" the change rather than preaching it.

"If you can't find your own words to express the idea or truth you know, then you might want to reconsider if you actually know it." Amen.

A Double Whammy, Part II

So yeah, I let my sensitivity get the better of me. My sister asked if I had mindlessly eaten because of the big picture fear/hurt/anger pain or the demeaned/stupid/rejected pain. I think it was both. And through that conversation with her, I was able to get even more clarity, which I will write about soon.

But now for Part II:

I took up training with kettlebells about a month ago. I asked Tim to take some photos of me working out. BIG MISTAKE! Or was it?

There I was, feeling all fit and strong, but when I looked at the photos, I cringed! Who was that fat, sweaty, grimacing, sneering woman?? It was as if all the love and acceptance I've worked so hard to feel for myself flew out the window in that one moment.

And then I realized that being honest with yourself is not the same as self-loathing. You can want to improve yourself without hating yourself but I haven't been able to separate the two! Or maybe it's just that I needed to work the self-love thing for a while before I could become more objective.

Have I been in serious denial? Have I let the whole body acceptance thing go too far and now it's taking the place of finding health and balance? I don't think so.

Part IV:
Total Acceptance

June 2010

"The privilege of a lifetime
is being who you are."
~ Joseph Campbell

What If?

What if I had a healthy relationship with food, exercise and my body? And what if I didn't make it about how much I weigh? And what if that relationship looked like this:

I eat when I'm hungry.

When I feel hunger it doesn't make me feel angry, sad, frustrated, or afraid.

I don't experience false hunger.

When I feel hunger, my first inclination is to stop and think, "hmmmm…what am I really hungry for? Do I need some protein?"

I automatically want what my body needs.

I never feel out of control.

I don't even have to think about control.

When I look in the mirror, I smile.

I don't binge. I have no desire to binge. In fact, I can't binge.

I am able to enjoy foods that I used to think were "bad."

I don't eat too much. I can't eat too much.

I love myself right now.

Loving myself is not dependent on the number on the scale, how many miles I ran, whether or not I worked out, or if I had a cookie instead of an apple

I don't think or worry about food.

I don't have to monitor myself.

I exercise because it makes me feel good.

I don't feel guilty if I miss a day...or a week.

I don't force myself.

I am gentle with myself.

I don't hurt myself.

I don't stress or obsess about what I "can" and "can't" eat.

I don't turn to food when I am sad/ happy/ frustrated/ tired/ annoyed/ frustrated/ giddy

I don't turn to food out of habit.

I am not deprived. I don't feel deprived.

And what if I felt this way not just for a day, for a week, for a month, but almost all the time?

And what if this is what I always believed to be possible but couldn't seem to figure out how to accomplish this miraculous feat?

And what if, one day, I realized that this was, in fact, how I've been living not just for a day, week or month, but several months?

It's rather shocking to me. I would sometimes have an hour or a day or two days at the most when I'd feel a modicum of peace and control around food and my body but it never lasted. And I've been hesitant to come out and say anything about what-is because I've wondered if it's a fluke.

I am not going to make this about weight loss because that's not really what it's about. It's about peace of mind and letting go. And the more peaceful I become, the more I am able let go. This also isn't about being perfect. I don't say this with an "it-will-never-happen-again-I-am-cured-hallelujah" sense of finality. I know better than that! It's an acknowledgement that I have reached what feels like a new "normal."

But, just for fun, what if, for the sake of argument, I did make it about weight for just a moment and said that my body is getting smaller and more toned, and that my clothes have become looser and in some cases too big?

It's Not Mine To Fix

"Evil is like a shadow - it has no real substance of its own,
it is simply a lack of light.
You cannot cause a shadow to disappear by trying to fight it, stamp
on it, by railing against it,
or any other form of emotional or physical resistance.
In order to cause a shadow to disappear,
you must shine light on it."
~ Shakti Gawain, teacher and author (1948-)

Over the past few days I've been tormented by something that has been a problem for many years. The gist of it (and this is something I figured out just now and am verbalizing for the first time) is that I have been trying to fix a relationship between two people I love - my husband and his daughter. And in doing so, I demonstrated that I didn't have respect for their feelings and that I didn't trust their ability to fix it themselves.

All these years I thought I was doing the right thing - the loving thing - even though I felt...dirty(?) every time I tried. Until this minute, I'd never made the connection as to why, but now I see it. I was not doing the loving thing, I was being selfish.

I'm a fixer from way back. I have a memory of my mother and father, before they were divorced, screaming at each other across the dining room table. And as children do, I internalized it as being my fault - that I wasn't "enough" for them to stay together, that I couldn't fix it. Of course, I don't believe that now, but it is what it is. And I have been trying to fix people ever since.

Just thinking about this reminds me of another time I thought I could fix something and it almost cost me one of the dearest relationships I have.

My sister and I are technically half siblings (we have the same father, but different mothers). She is nine years younger than I am, and we didn't grow up in the same household, but as far as I am concerned, we are sisters in every sense of the word. I can't imagine my life without her.

Several years ago, I did something stupid and selfish that threatened our relationship. We didn't talk for months. It was one of the most painful times in my life and it happened because I didn't like myself much at the time and because I didn't know how to be loving without also being critical and judgmental. This is how I treated myself, as well.

It was our father's wife Barbara who prompted me to reach out, apologize, and mend the rift. I am sure I would have done the right thing eventually, but it was Barbara who gently prodded me to take action. And what's interesting is that by the time I reached out to my sister to make amends, I had also reached out to myself and had begun to lose weight. I just now, this very minute, made that connection.

But many, many years ago, before my sister was even born, there was another incident that threatened our relationship. I can only tell this story from the bits and pieces I have heard from various (but not all) sources, and not from the perspective of having been there and witnessing it, because I was only a small child. I am not sure if I have all the facts, and I am certain that cannot speak from any other perspective than my own.

My parents divorced when I was three and both remarried when I was six. My mother and stepfather, at the urging of the minister who married them, approached my father and suggested that it would be in my best interest if he gave up his parental rights, never saw me again, and allowed my stepfather to adopt and raise me. In return, he would no longer have to pay child support. I am not sure if they offered him an additional incentive.

My father has since told me that he wasn't sure what he should do. I know he wanted to do the right thing, as did my mother. In the end, it was my stepmother (my sister's mother) who did the right thing for me and said "absolutely not."

I can't pretend to understand how this affected everyone else, either negatively or positively. All I know is that if my stepmother hadn't stood up for me (and my father), my sister and I wouldn't be sisters.

When I told her that I was writing about this, she wondered what it would have been like to discover, years later, that she had a sister she didn't know. We talked about what it must be like for the many families who have endured these kinds of separations and secrets, only to find out the truth years later.

And who knows what kind of relationship I'd have with my father, if at all. Would I have eventually gone looking for him? Would he look for me? These are the kinds of questions we ask ourselves when we think back to those pivotal decisions and those defining moments. Except in my case, in this particular situation, it wasn't up to me.

You might wonder what any of this has to do with weight loss or why I am sharing it, but this is part of the journey. It is with the loving acknowledgment of past hurts, of our own mistakes, that we are able to live lighter.

The World Peace Diet*

*Just kidding...I don't really mean "diet."

I spent this past weekend with approximately 400 women at a retreat led by Geneen Roth, author of <u>Women Food And God</u>. You can not read this book and not be changed by it, whether you have issues with food or not.

The overarching message I got from the retreat was:

When we begin to love ourselves, we begin to do the work of world peace.

I don't care if I sound like a beauty pageant contestant or a hippie...

I have written about this before, but not quite in this way. I believe that:

...the more I fill myself up with what I love to do (and writing is one of those things)...

...the more I look inward to understand myself...

...the more I do this...

...then the more I love myself and the healthier I become.

AND:

...the more I love myself and the healthier I become, the better I am in my relationships and the more love I have to give.

It's like I've become a love generator. Love, turned inward, multiplies so there's more to give! Love is infinite...it creates itself. The more I love, the more I love.

So you can see where this is going, right?

Let's look at what's going on in the world. We've got wars, terrorism, propaganda. We've got this side threatening that side. We've got this guy wanting to burn that guy's holy book. So we fight for change because we don't know any other way. And the basic ingrained lesson is, war works.

Now let's look at what was going on with me. I had an unhealthy relationship with food and with myself, not to mention a few members of my family. I overate. I was not as healthy as I could be. I would sometimes hurt myself by exercising too much. I felt broken. And I thought the only way to change was to struggle and fight for it...that there was no way that it would come easily and naturally. I thought I had take on other people's goals. I thought I had to live by other people's rules. And because I didn't have any other way of seeing it, the basic ingrained lesson was, war works. And as I write this I think of all the war-like analogies in the diet/weight loss culture: boot camp, challenge, victory, battle, conquer, fight, loser, winner...

My body, my weight, and my *self* were a microcosm of the ingrained lesson that the only way to change is through shame, guilt, hate, and deprivation.

I don't know exactly when I decided to step away from the diet-binge war but a key moment in the process was when I decided to stop weighing myself because it was just too damn painful to get on that scale. Another moment was when I learned how to practice acceptance right this minute no matter what. And then there was the moment that I realized that I can just *be* with exuberance and grief, love and rage, jealousy and confidence, insecurity and comfort, pettiness and generosity...I can *be* with all of it without having to numb myself.

And there's been a million other moments.

It's been a continuous letting go. And now it's an active reminder that world peace starts with me.

If Only Needy And Desperate
Were Attractive Qualities

What are you really hungry for?

I've been asking myself that question for years. Oprah has asked it. Geneen Roth has asked it. And I am sure countless others have asked it.

And so I've been answering:

- I am hungry to write
- I am hungry to be heard
- I am hungry for acknowledgement
- I am hungry to be seen

SEE ME!!!

And so when I showed up at Kripalu for the "Women Food And God" retreat I was all in a dither. I felt like I might just jump out of my skin! I was so excited to meet Geneen because I wanted to thank her for not only reading my blog, but for Tweeting about it!! I told a few of the women I met when I arrived about it. We saw her in the Kripalu dining room and they encouraged me to approach her.

Inside I felt like a jerk...like a little kid or a groupie or something. I have always disdained people who approach celebrities/authority figures and fawn all over them. And inside, not so deep down, I knew this is what I would be doing if I approached her. And so I didn't...but I was still scheming.

If I could just come up with the absolute right thing to say, it would be okay and Geneen would see me and hear me and acknowledge me and tell me I am okay. In fact, she'd call me up in front of the entire retreat and tell everyone about me.

BWAHAHAHAHAHAHAHAHA!!!

This has been the story of my life since I can remember! And it's so embarrassing to admit! I am so fucking needy and I crave attention from those whom I believe can bestow...I don't even know what...on me. And even though I just laughed out loud, now I am crying because I am ashamed that I feel this way...that I have this need. But at the same time, I know I am okay, too.

And here's the thing. After a while I realized what was going on and that I didn't need any outside acknowledgment. I have everything I need. I don't need her or anyone else to tell me I am okay. And so I relaxed, let go of that need, and soaked up the wisdom of all the women around me, including her.

And on that note, I want to explain how I create love for myself. You know that googly feeling you get when you see a baby or a kitten or a puppy? That tender, melty, feeling? And you know how it can actually become a physical sensation? Practice being able to bring that feeling up in yourself and then turn it inward. Soften your eyes, take some slow, deep breaths. Then do it while looking at yourself in the mirror. Then do it naked if you can. The more you do this, the easier it becomes.

There is actual scientific proof that doing this improves breast health, according to Dr. Christiane Northrup, and so it wouldn't surprise me if it also improved the health of our entire body.

I had the opportunity to interview Dr. Northrup in 2007 for a local magazine prior to her speaking at a women's conference sponsored by a local hospital. Her talked was entitled "Becoming An Exceptional Woman While Remaining Human: 10 Principles For Health and Happiness." I asked her to give me a preview of what she was going to say.

"I am going to provide a whole new way for women to think about their health and their bodies...that it's more pleasurable and fun than they think. The old expression 'no pain no gain' only produces more pain."

She went on to say that she believes we women have "enormous power" in our bodies and that it can be used to heal.

"The first step is to understand that your thoughts are translated through your emotions and that your emotions physically affect your tissues, for better or for worse. So the path to good health is through pleasure not pain. I will also be talking specifically about how thoughts and emotions affect your heart. The electromagnetic field of your heart is created by your emotions and beliefs...and they profoundly affect your health and circumstances."

So developing those googly feelings actually does something physiologically. It relaxes us. It's tranquil. And when we're tranquil, we're not stressed, and when we're not stressed, our bodies are not over-producing the fight-or-flight hormone cortisol, which is known to have such negative effects as increased abdominal fat, higher blood pressure, lower immunity and inflammatory responses in the body.

So yeah, there's science to back up the woo-woo. Remember the chapter about neural plasticity and dendrites?

Needy And Desperate, Part II

Imagine a sneering, disgusted, demoralizing voice:

You pathetic idiot!!

Who do you think you are??

I didn't hear The Voice right away, but as yesterday afternoon wore on I started to feel shamed. I was breathing more shallowly, I felt slightly panicked. My shoulders were hunched and I felt tight and constricted.

You're running around desperately trying to get someone's, anyone's attention with your pathetic drivel.

Look at you, wasting all that time online, calling attention to yourself. You've got nothing to offer so just stop it!!

Go away you spoiled brat.

The Voice got louder and louder and I got more needy and desperate.

The need to be seen and heard was at a fever pitch and I was going from forum to forum talking about my "success" and my blog, trampling all over Geneen Roth's Facebook page, leaving preachy comments on other people's blogs…doing the one thing I've been striving not to do. I was in I've-got-it-all-figured-out-so-you-better-listen-to-me mode.

I felt like I was a little kid, jumping up and down, waving her arms saying, ooooh oooh me me me!! Look at me!! I couldn't help myself!

I was in binge mode, but not with food!

You don't deserve to be noticed, your efforts are pathetic. You don't have an original thought in your head, you're just parroting others, riding their coat tails and thinking you're all that.

Today is a new day. Today is a clearer day. I understand myself. I know what I want. I want to be me, not Geneen Roth. I want what I have, not what she has.

You're Not The Boss Of Me

That is how I disengaged from The Voice yesterday.

Shut UP! Just shut the fuck up!

It's what Geneen Roth suggested we do when we hear The Voice. Disengaging from it may take different forms at different times, depending on a number of factors. If, as a child, you weren't allowed to express anger, then an angry tone is a good tone to use.

If you you're feeling the need for a little tenderness, than perhaps a more soothing tone is needed:

"I'm sorry, but you can't talk to me that way. I understand that you're scared and that you're just trying to protect me, but you're not helping. There there... you'll be fine, just hold my hand and we'll do this together."

Or maybe a little humor works:

"You've got to be kidding me...do you think I'm that gullible?"

An exercise we did during the retreat involved writing down two decisions that we made about ourselves when we were children and the ways in which our relationship with food addressed and advanced those decisions. In many ways it was similar to the work I did in the Living Lighter classes from Parts I and II.

Here's what I wrote:

"I'm a spoiled brat. And because of that decision, I hid myself so as not to get too much attention, to not shine too brightly, because then not only would I be a spoiled brat, I'd be a spoiled brat that was showing off. I hid by using food...and got fat because we all know it's impossible for fat people to shine."

And that right there ladies and gentlemen is why The Voice has been so loud over the past few days.

Now that I've gotten a little clarity, I can easily see the difference between the *"here I am and I am so happy to be me"* me and the *"I am needy and desperate so please pay attention to me"* me.

And what I understand is that when I am being the *"here I am and I am so happy to be me"* me, I am authentic and I feel good inside, physically and emotionally. I respond from a place of love.

When I am being the *"I am needy and desperate so please pay attention to me"* me, I disregard my intuition and I respond from a place of envy and hate. Thus the frantic bingeing behavior (although it was not food on which I binged).

Oh The Stories I Have Told

I used to tell stories – sometimes based on the truth (but embellished) and other times outright lies. Some of these lies were funny and relatively benign – "I was born on an airplane" – but other times they were destructive, not at all funny – "I was raped." And everything in between.

I'm not sure when I started telling stories but I continued up until about 10 years ago. I understand now why I told them…I thought they would make me more attractive, funny, interesting, tragic, relatable, dramatic, loveable.

I've come clean with the most important people in my life about these lies, so this isn't a confession. And just so you know I haven't lied or embellished the truth in this book. What I have done is told my version of stories. We all do that.

Some recent experiences have me reflecting on the phenomenon. I know I've heard this before…it's not a new concept, but let me lay it out for you the way I understand it:

There's what happened.

Then there's the story I tell about what happened.

And finally there's the story I tell about what it means that it happened, and how I feel about it.

I am not saying that the stories anyone tells about what happened, or about how they feel about what happened, are lies...but that they are perceptions and not complete, objective "reality."

So yeah, I've been thinking about this a lot lately and I thought it was worth exploring here because I realize that it's the stories I tell about what happened and what they mean, that weigh me down.

For example, there's the story of my first marriage. I married a guy from Brazil...a guy I met in a bar just four months prior to marrying. He needed a Green Card. I had convinced myself that he really loved me even though, if I am really honest, I knew he didn't. The marriage was sham on all levels. I felt forced to divorce him because he was not what I considered a willing participant in the marriage. I was angry but I portrayed myself as a victim and told anyone who would listen that he took complete and total advantage of me, leaving me heartbroken, in debt...and feeling like an utter fool.

I declared bankruptcy a few years after my divorce and my story is that I was forced to because of the "tax burden" he left for me. That's partially the truth, but the bigger part of the truth is that I spent more money that I was making.

Then there's the story about why I was so desperate and lacking self-esteem that I would enter in to such a marriage in the first place. Was my story "because my parents got divorced when I was three"? Or how about, "I grew up in a dysfunctional family"? Or maybe just because?? Maybe that's just the way it was supposed to work out for me.

Another example: someone claimed to have slept with a former boyfriend of mine (after we had broken up), even though said former boyfriend said it never happened. The story I told after the fact was designed, not to elicit sympathy for me, but to elicit disgust for the someone...to "build my case" against that person.

And another: I was out of the country just before 9/11 and arrived at JFK Airport at 9/9. On the morning of 9/11, Tim had to fly to Virginia for work. He flew out of Providence, RI, into Regan National in Washington, DC, where he made a connecting flight to Norfolk, just 15 minutes before the Pentagon was hit. He was in the air while planes were crashing into the World Trade Center. Even though what was happening scared the crap out of me, I knew he was okay. But in the days, months, and for several years afterwards, when I told the story, I would tell it in a more evocative way. It was the truth, but it became more dramatic in the telling than it actually was.

And what about the rape story? That's a doozy. I had sex for the first time at a pretty young age but to this day I do not count it as losing my virginity and I choose not to reveal why in order to protect the innocent. Afterwards I thought I might be pregnant so I made up a rather unlikely story about being raped by a faceless, nameless, unrecognizable man, just in case. What's ironic is that I didn't tell anyone the rape story until well after I knew that I wasn't pregnant. I didn't "need" the story, but I "used" it. And what's destructive about the story is that I often concluded it by saying that it (the rape) didn't affect me or damage me in any way.

I could go on and on, but you get the picture. These are the stories I've told myself and others...stories that made me feel better about myself, stories that helped me feel right, stories that helped me feel like I was getting revenge. I got off on these stories. They gave me an out and allowed me to abdicate responsibility.

What I see is that I made a whole series of decisions, then came up with stories and lies to make myself feel better, but which really led to a lot of physical, emotional, and mental heaviness. In fact, I'd go as far as to say that these stories took me farther away from who I really am. And the farther I got, the "heavier" I got.

As I said, anyone who knows me really well already knows the truth and it's been quite a while since I've even felt the need to tell an outright lie. But I recognize that I'm still telling stories about what happened...mostly in an effort to understand.

> *"Whenever two people meet,*
> *there are really six people present.*
> *There is each man as he sees himself,*
> *each man as the other person sees him,*
> *and each man as he really is."*
> ~ William James, pragmatist, philosopher, and psychologist
> (1842 - 1910)

This whole weight loss thing has turned into my quest to figure out how to bring "who I really am" as close as possible to "how I see myself" and to "how others see me."

"Honest" is way up there on the list.

From What-If To What-Is

Remember the "what if" chapter? I want to explain, as best I can, how I think I went from "what if" to "what is." This is a unique and personal set of circumstances and not a "how-to" or "10 steps to perfection" type of deal. I don't believe in that.

I started feeling my feelings, embracing the good, the bad, the ugly. Saying it out loud. I learned that "going there" isn't as scary and painful as NOT "going there."

I learned what self-acceptance is and started practicing it on a regular basis.

I am able to look at myself naked in the mirror and feel tremendous love and respect for myself.

I learned that I have everything I need, inside myself.

I stopped beating myself up (mostly).

I understand (finally!) that self-hated does not lead to positive change! You can't hate yourself to thinness or health!

I actively decided not to view my health/weight/body as a struggle or battle.

I let go of numbers and other specific measurements.

I opened my mind to other ways of being. I became a learner instead of a know-it-all. Resistant Karen is not so resistant any more.

I stopped setting goals attached to weight.

I don't drink as much as I used to. This was a tough one, and I've written about it several times. But I think it's helped in regulating my appetite, carb cravings and false hunger. I feel somewhat disingenuous writing this because the choice to stop drinking was sort of made for me. I am not sure what has happened, but my body does not respond well to more than a glass of wine. In fact, it doesn't respond well to sugar (and that's what alcohol is...sugar). If that were not the case, I am not sure I'd be writing this. And writing this is a good example of me "going there"...going to a place that is uncomfortable.

So yeah, going to those dark places and shining a light in the darkest corners, while uncomfortable, is ultimately how I got the darkness to disappear. It doesn't mean that my life if perfect. Every day is not happy-happy-joy-joy. I have bad days. I cry. I get angry. Sometimes I even have panic attacks. But now I understand that these things won't destroy me and so I am not as afraid as I once was. And now that I am not as afraid, I don't have to numb myself.

From Either/Or To Both/And

I am sitting here wearing a top that used to be too tight through the chest/back and a skirt that used to pull through the hips and pinched at the waist. I honestly didn't think I'd ever be able to comfortably wear these items again, and I was honestly okay with that.

It's funny because I recently cleaned out my closet and got rid of everything that didn't fit me, whether too big or too small. But I kept a few favorite things (both too big and too small) and now I'm glad I did.

I've written a lot about struggling and how I don't want to struggle with my body. Here's what I usually say: "if I view this as a struggle...as a fight to be fought, then that's exactly what I'll get."

I believe that. I want it to be easy. I want it to come naturally. I resist the idea that a healthy body is or should be a struggle. I know in the deepest part of myself that this is the way it should be. I sense that there are skeptics out there...heck, even I'm skeptical sometimes. We need proof! We need before and after pictures! We need numbers and measurements! We need goals and challenges!

And so I am sitting here, in clothes I didn't think I'd ever wear again, feeling...what? A little shocked, for sure. Smug? Not really...well maybe a little, but knowing that smug doesn't get me anywhere! I definitely feel triumphant and proud. I am doing it my way! (And for as long as I can remember, I've confounded others, and myself, because I just can't seem to follow the rules when it comes to stuff like this.)

But if I am honest, can I look back at the past year-plus and say that I haven't struggled? NO!

I didn't want to struggle over counting calories and worrying about every bite I put into my mouth. I didn't want to struggle with the number on the scale. I didn't want to struggle with a timetable. I didn't want to struggle with hunger.

But I was willing to struggle with my emotions and (certain) relationships. I was willing to struggle with certain aspects of my health. I was willing to struggle with having patience for myself. And I was willing to struggle with finding my own way. And so I put the scale away, decided to trust myself (and we all know how hard it is trust ourselves, our bodies, when it feels like we've been betrayed so many times before!), and to have the patience to let it take as much time as it needed to take.

I read an article by Martha Beck called "How To Solve a Thorny Problem," in O magazine (July 2010 issue) and it discusses the idea that, when it comes to yes-or-no dilemmas, the most powerful thing you can ask is, what if both answers are true?

She uses the example of a woman who has met a new guy who appears to be both a player AND a thoughtful guy who really seems to like her. And a friend asks her, "What if both things are true?"

It's called "both-and" thinking (versus "either-or" thinking).

So what if both embracing struggle and resisting struggle is the right answer? What if struggle is both good and bad? And how do you know when to embrace it and when to resist it? I don't have a definitive answer for all, but I will say that I must have instinctually known when it was right to struggle and when it was right to let go.

Beck calls it a duel-emma, a situation that leads to two true, but apparently contradictory conclusions. And how are we supposed to move forward? Beck says the only way out is to use a statement that draws attention to it. In other words, awareness. "It takes you beyond the two choices you thought you had. It opens up previously unseen possibilities and opportunities," she says.

So, for me, in the past I thought I had two choices: either struggle with those things I didn't want to struggle with (and be unhappy), or be fat (and be unhappy). Somewhere along the way I started (without realizing it) using both-and thinking...and a whole lot of wonderful possibilities and opportunities have come my way...possibilities and opportunities that I never imagined.

A Karmic Bitch Slap

OR

A Chapter In Which I Express My Anger Constructively...

In Which I Ask Myself How I Really Feel...

In Which I Practice Just Feeling My Feelings

I went to see my hormone specialist. It's been a little more than three months since I started this new regimen. I'd had more blood work and saliva tests done to see where things stood.

But first of all, I have to say that I feel so much better, physically, mentally, and emotionally, than I have in a long while and I believe that getting my hormones back into balance is the main reason. It remains to be seen if Lyme is an issue, and I am beginning to wonder if I really had it at all. But I digress...

I told him about how great I am feeling, that I am exercising more, that I've lost inches off my waist, that I am wearing clothes that once didn't fit, etc. I told him that my cravings and "false hunger" have been greatly reduced, and so on.

The results of my tests showed that everything has improved, except my cholesterol and my thyroid function. In fact, my cholesterol has gotten worse (the overall number went up, as did the LDL (or "bad") number, and the particle size pattern of my LDL cholesterol has gone from large and buoyant, to small and dense). My HDL and triglycerides are fine.

I guess this is no surprise, given that I stopped taking Lipitor. He suggested that all of this could be due to the fact that my thyroid still isn't where it needs to be. He suggested a thyroid hormone that is effective and which also happens to help weight-loss.

Then he switched gears and said that he had a colleague who had recently lost 35 pounds...how the guy had been working out like crazy for months and hadn't been able to lose a pound but then BAM, he lost weight. At first I thought he was talking about the thyroid hormone, but then he picked up a brochure, handed it to me, and started talking about some new program. On the cover of the brochure it said "Ideal Protein, Your Last Diet."

::::::insert sound of screeching brakes::::::

NO! No diets! No programs! NO NO NO! Don't you get it?? I am trying to trust myself here. Don't you DARE try and sell me a diet!!

Okay, that's not what I said to him. But that's what I was thinking.

He went on to say that it's a program that teaches you how to eat certain types of foods at the same time, and how you shouldn't eat carbs and fats in the same meal, and about getting more protein, blah blah blah. I tried to get him to tell me specifics, like is it actual meals that you buy? He mentioned that he was going to have an informational presentation at his office so he can learn more about it and he said he was inviting interested patients.

I tried to tell him, as briefly as I could, about where I've been in my life and why the last thing I want to do now is "go on a diet." He said that this wasn't a diet. I asked him again what they were selling and I got the impression that it was protein in the form of various products like shakes, bars, chips and so on. He said that it involves eating "your own food" but he also said that on this program, you end up eating about 800 calories a day.

And here's the thing, I got the impression, as he was telling me about it, that he was expecting me to light up with glee and excitement, as if I'd just discovered the Holy Grail of weight loss and would immediately and desperately sign up for it.

Here's the part where I practice:

I feel upset, angry and betrayed. It makes me not want to trust this doctor who I really want to trust! I know that he knows his stuff and is highly respected. He's been voted, many times, as a top doctor in our state. I'm mad because I feel like I have to defend the fact that I am seeing him.

DEEEEEEP BREATH

I feel rebellious and like stamping my foot and saying, "you can't make me." I feel like eating something "bad" just to spite him. Not really, but sort of.

DEEEEEP BREATH
UNSCRUNCHING SHOULDERS

I feel like society has gotten to the point where, if you don't want to "lose 3-7 pounds per week," you're the weird one...

DEEEEEP BREATH

UNSCRUNCHING SHOULDERS

SOFTENING EYES

I am okay, and he's okay too. It's not like he wants to feed me poison. Maybe he just hasn't had a patient like me. Maybe he's under pressure from his other patients to help them lose weight more quickly. Perhaps this program will help some people.

DEEEEEP BREATH

UNSCRUNCHING SHOULDERS

SOFTENING EYES

ACKNOWLEDGING REALITY

I feel better, and am doing better...and I know better. And I will continue to see this doctor because he is helping me. I am an intelligent, adult woman who can make her own decisions. I am okay.

But not really.

I feel frantic and confused and overwhelmed.

I feel like my desire to trust myself is being tested.

I can't concentrate on anything.

I am jumping from one thing to another and not finishing anything.

It feels like things are spinning out of control.

I can't get centered.

I need to be soothed and told that everything will be okay.

I feel like a bad girl.

I feel like when I am hungry, I won't be giving myself what my body needs because I am a fool who thought she knew what she was doing but obviously doesn't.

How could I have made SO much progress and then feel like it's nothing? Maybe I am just imagining that my clothes fit better.

That doctor planted so much doubt in my head!

I hate that. What does that mean about who I am? My character?

It makes me angrier than it should. Why can't I just let it go? Why does my reaction feel over-blown? Or maybe it's not, but I am so freaking out of touch that I have no clue.

Or maybe, in my desire to trust myself, I am deluding myself? Looking for a way to get out of doing what's right for me?

Why is it so threatening to me that this doctor asked me to consider this program and lose 20 pounds?

It makes me realize that it's damned hard to trust myself. Why is that?

It all seems so complex and so simple at the same time.

Why can't I just feel angry without all this guilt?

I feel like I'm a bad girl.
I feel like I'm a bad girl.
I feel like I'm a bad girl.
I feel like I'm a bad girl.
I feel like I'm a bad girl.
I feel like I'm a bad girl.

Everyone is looking at me in pity and they are laughing because they can see what I can't.

Part Of The Process

The previous chapter was an exercise in being with emotions that felt as if they could destroy me. In the moment of writing, I was crying, sobbing even, and it felt uncomfortable. But it also felt fantastic. I was not destroyed.

The whole situation presented me with an opportunity. My first reaction is to say that I am being given an opportunity to prove him wrong, but that's an old pattern, based on old ways of being.

And what about all that "bad girl" talk? What was that about?

I think it, too, goes back to old patterns and ways of being.

"Don't talk back."

"Listen to me when I talk to you."

"Don't rock the boat."

"I know what's best for you."

But there's something else. Even though I haven't weighed myself in over a year, I know I've lost some weight. I've lost a few inches off my waist (yes, I am still measuring, even though I haven't mentioned it) and am wearing clothes that used to be too tight. In the past five or six months, the false hunger and cravings have gone away. That kind of "control" is something I am still getting used to.

And maybe that's what's bothering me...he didn't recognize this, even when I told him.

Whatever Works, Right?

At the basis of what I've been doing in this book is a desire…a desire for what?

Thinness? Happiness? Healthiness? Fitness? Peace? Contentment? Acceptance? Confidence? Normalcy? Control? To weigh X? To wear size X? All of the above? Forever and ever?

Is there a right way to get "all of the above forever and ever." Some advocate intuitive/mindful eating, some swear by a certain "diet," and others believe in counting calories or points. And don't forget exercise!

But here's the thing: if what you're doing works for you, why change it? I think the answer lies in the definition of "works" and that definition is going to be different depending with whom you speak.

For some, "works" means they've put their noses to the grind stone, counted calories, exercised, reached their goal weight, and have kept the weight off for a certain amount of time.

For others, "works" means they're healthy, they feel good in their clothes, they can look in the mirror without cringing (in fact, when they do look in the mirror, they smile and think loving thoughts), and they don't "obsess" about food or the number on the scale.

And then there's everything in between (not that I think the two examples I've provided are polar opposites... they're just two examples). I pretty much fall into the second category.

I have always wanted to believe that this was possible, "this" being feeling good about my body (no matter what), losing weight, and being healthy WITHOUT having to weigh myself, diet, count calories, and feel hungry. It's taken me a damned long time to figure it out for myself, but I did. And I get that it may not be what "works" for someone else.

I think one of the hardest lessons to learn is that we can know something but not be able to live it...have knowledge but not know how to apply it. It is possible; it just takes time, patience, and practice. As I like to say, "it takes as long as it needs to take." If we force ourselves to fake it before we're really able to live it and know it in our cells, then we might slide back...but even THAT is part of the process too. It's part of the practice. The problem is we see it as "failure" instead. And we all know what happens when we think we've failed...

But here's the real test of whether it "works": no matter which category (or subset, or combination thereof) you want to put yourself in, are you truly happy and confident in being there? Do you trust yourself?? Do you worry about what others think?

I sometimes do. I like where I am right now but there are times when I think that others are judging me. Although I SAY I don't obsess about the number on the scale, the fact is I don't even know what it is because I don't want to know. I haven't weighed myself in over a year. And that in and of itself might be considered obsessing or unhealthy. But for now, it's what "works" for me.

Revisiting Insanity

Remember when I wrote this?

"The definition of insanity is doing the same thing over and over again and expecting different results." – Albert Einstein

And you know what? I realize that this is exactly what I've been doing: eating the same old, same old, and expecting to lose weight. I had cut back and begun making better choices, but it was only enough to stop me from gaining. It wasn't enough to lose weight!

As I read this I realized that what I failed to realize at the time was that the "insanity" had nothing to do (at least not directly) with what I was or wasn't eating, but rather with the pattern in which I was stuck:

I am broken and need to fix myself.

If I could just figure out the magic formula and then stick to it forever, I'd lose weight and then I'd be happier.

It's just a matter of controlling and restricting myself.

I'd been in this same pattern for so long and I'd held these same beliefs for so long and yet I expected different results.

Now, while I understand that restriction, dieting, and focusing on "losing weight" works for some people, so far in my life, it hasn't, at least not long term. And that's what I want: long-term, sustainable results WITHOUT constantly feeling stressed, worried, panicky, or desperate. I understand that feeling stressed, worried, panicky, or desperate ONCE IN A WHILE is normal and okay and maybe even necessary! But not on a daily basis...not as a primary way of being. Besides, there are plenty of other reasons and opportunities for stressed-worried-panicky-desperate...

And so I got sane. I broke out of the I-need-to-fix-myself pattern and stopped holding the if-I-could-only-lose-weight-I'd-be-happy beliefs.

Something else that occurred to me recently is that since I have found sanity, my motivation has changed. I used to be addicted to the reactions of others. I was all about someone else saying, "wow you look great" or "how much weight have you lost?" or "how did you do it?"

In fact I recently had an appointment with my naturopath and when she saw me she said "wow, you've lost some weight...you look great!" I'm not going to lie and say that I didn't like it that she noticed, because I did...but only because it validated that getting sane works!

Besides, what I really wanted to know was whether or not my cholesterol had improved even though I am no longer taking a statin drug (it had)! I have faith that it will continue to improve, even without medication. I truly believe that part of the reason is because I am not beating myself up and, as a result, am not putting as much stress on my body and psyche as I used to. I haven't restricted any particular foods, I haven't told myself that I can't have this or that.

"What we see depends mainly on what we look for."
~Sir John Lubbock

Now that I feel whole and okay-as-is, I have a whole different perspective. What I see now is completely different than what I saw a year ago because I am looking for something different.

How Does This Book End?

So here I am at the end of the book. This is the last chapter.

When I started writing, I believed that "before" equals all that is negative, unhappy, fat, and unhealthy, and that "after" equals all that is positive, happy, thin, and healthy. First you're *here*, then you're *there* and everything is perfect.

I believed that at this point I'd be "thin" and "beautiful" and "toned." I believed that I'd have "a perfect body." I believed that I would have achieved a "healthy weight."

And that's it. That's all I could imagine. That's what I believed would be the only acceptable end to this story. I was afraid that if that *wasn't* true at the end of the book, then I would have somehow failed. Failed you and failed myself.

Being a weight loss success story is tough. The "after" photo, that one moment in time, is captured and it's supposed to represent happily ever after. You reach that moment and you stay that weight forever and ever. But we all know that's not the case. Our weight bounces up and down, sometimes it goes lower than the "goal weight" and sometimes it goes higher. Much higher. But are we not still a success?

I have spent enough time being afraid.

First I was afraid that I'd never lose weight (even though I wasn't actively trying). Then I was afraid (when I WAS actively trying and losing) that I wouldn't reach my goal weight. *Then –*

because I never did reach it – I was afraid of what other people thought of me. Then I was afraid that I'd gain the weight back (which I did). And then I was afraid that I wouldn't be able to lose the weight I had regained.

And all that fear kept building on itself until I started to shine a light on it. And that's when I started writing.

And now, here I am. Happier and less afraid than I've ever been. Here's what else I've learned along the way:

"Going there" isn't as scary and painful as NOT "going there."

I do not define myself by how much I weigh, nor by how much weight I've gained or lost.

I eat when I'm hungry. If I eat when I am not hungry, I notice it.

When I feel hunger, it doesn't make me feel angry, sad, frustrated, or afraid.

I don't feel out of control.

I don't panic when I feel hungrier than "normal."

I am able to enjoy foods that I used to think were "bad."

I find it difficult to eat too much.

I love myself *right now*.

I am able to look at myself naked in the mirror and feel tremendous love and respect for my body and myself.

Loving myself isn't dependent on whether or not I worked out, or if I had a cookie instead of an apple.

I do not view my health/weight/body as a struggle or battle.

I stopped beating myself up.

I opened my mind to other ways of being. I became a learner instead of a know-it-all. Resistant Karen is not so resistant any more.

I don't worry about food. I don't monitor myself around food. I am aware, not obsessed.

I don't feel guilty if I miss a day…or a week…of exercise.

I don't force myself. I am gentle with myself. I don't hurt myself.

I don't stress or obsess about what I "can" and "can't" eat.

I don't turn to food when I am sad/happy/tired/annoyed/frustrated/giddy.

I don't turn to food out of habit.

I am not deprived. I don't *feel* deprived.

I stopped setting goals attached to weight.

I feel this way not just for a day, for a week, or for a month, but almost all the time.

When I operate from a place of acceptance (not fear), I automatically do better in all areas my life: my relationships are better, I write better, I eat better, I take care of myself better. I give better.

This isn't about perfection. I don't say this with an "it-will-never-happen-again-I-am-cured-hallelujah" sense of finality. I know better than that!

I understand that it took as long as it needed to take.

I understand that I don't always know what progress looks like, and that progress sometimes looks like something I wish it didn't.

I no longer have a "goal weight." I haven't weighed myself in over a year. My goals are respect, awareness, truth, trust, and presence.

So take a deeeeeep belly breath and say it with me: "I am fine with who I am right this very minute. I love my body right now. I will love my body in the next minute and the next minute after that. And in the next hour and the next day. No matter what."

And guess what? It's true! I have the perfect body for me. Right this very minute, my body is absolute perfection.

I know you know this, but I'll say it anyway: the journey never ends and "after" is just an illusion.

A Final Note:
First Comes Love

"We cannot change anything until we accept it. Condemnation does not liberate, it oppresses.
~ Carl Jung

Yeah, I know it sounds woo woo, but in the healthy body business, I believe love MUST come first. It's why I started my blog two years ago. It was like an experiment. I wanted to see if I could love myself to thinness. Or something like that.

There are theories that suggest it's possible. The paradoxical theory of change states: *"change occurs when one becomes what he is, not when he tries to become what he is not. Change does not take place through a coercive attempt by the individual or by another person to change him, but it does take place if one takes the time and effort to be what he is -- to be fully invested in his current positions. By rejecting the role of change agent, we make meaningful and orderly change possible."*

My experience has shown this to be true. And it led me down an unexpected path. When I first started writing two years ago, I just wanted to lose weight and stop hating my body, in that order.

Mostly I looked inside at emotional issues and in doing so, discovered a lot more than I bargained for. But mostly what I discovered is that at root of all healing is love. Love – not "stop hating" – has to come first.

Let's start with this premise:

What if being sick makes you fat and not the other way around? And what it the reason you *"eat too much"* or *"can't control yourself"* or *"feel hungry all the time"* has nothing to do (at least not directly) with emotions and is not a character flaw (like so many of us were brought up to believe)? Or what if the reason you can't lose weight and *keep it off without a <u>struggle</u>* has to do with a physical imbalance?

Ten+ years ago:
- I weighed ~225 pounds.
- I didn't exercise (or if I did, it was sporadic).
- I was a binge eater (carbs, fat).
- I walked around with a cloud of self-doubt over my head.
- I was on a statin medication to control my cholesterol.
- I was on birth control pills and had been for 15 years.
- I "wanted to lose weight" and had "tried" many times, but it "didn't work."

Five years ago:
- In an effort to once again "try to lose weight" I started a relatively new type of therapy called Emotional Freedom Technique. It was through EFT that I realized that I had been walking around full of self-loathing and without any self-confidence or self-acceptance.
- Seemingly, the stars aligned and through EFT I found myself wanting to do the "right" things for myself, health-wise.
- I started exercising.
- I counted calories and tracked the ratios of protein, carbohydrates, and fat.

- I lost 55 pounds over the course of 18 months.
- I remained on the statin medication, because even though I had lost weight and was exercising regularly, my cholesterol went back up when I tried weaning myself from the medication.
- I remained on birth control pills, even though my husband had a vasectomy, because it was "easier" and because my doctor didn't see any reason to stop.
- I'd had my gallbladder out.
- I didn't feel comfortable with myself.
- I didn't trust myself around food.
- I was disappointed and ashamed because, even though I had lost 55 pounds, I hadn't reached my "goal weight" (which would have required losing 76 pounds).

Two years ago:
- I'd regained half the weight I had lost.
- I was once again "depressed" and full of shame.
- I was still on birth control pills.
- I was still on the statin medication.
- My body hurt.
- I found it hard to exercise, but pushed myself anyway because I had to somehow control the weight.
- I found myself "white-knuckling" it around food.
- It seemed that I was hungry all the time.
- Being hungry made me feel guilty, resentful and angry.
- I was tired of trying so damned hard!

One year ago:
- I had been practicing self-acceptance again (and realizing that it is indeed practice, not something you get once and can forget about).
- I decided to see a naturopathic physician in my area. I thought she might help me lose weight.
- Really? I thought there might be a magic pill!
- She recommended stopping the birth control pills, which I did right away.
- She wanted to get me off the statin medication, but recommended waiting to address other issues first.
- The other issues included Lyme disease, Epstein Barr virus, hormone imbalance, thyroid imbalance, adrenal imbalance, and deficiency in certain vitamins, minerals and nutrients.
- She told me that no, I was not just a lazy slob who couldn't control herself and had no willpower.

With the naturopath's help, along with that of a hormone specialist, my body came in to balance. For the first time...ever? I know what a balanced body feels like! I understand that my body is a holistic system, not a mass of individual symptoms that need to be masked or suppressed.

And so today:
- I am 48 years old.
- Although I am not focused on "losing weight" I am.
- I have lost six inches from my waist in the past year and my body is more toned.
- I exercise less than I used to and my body doesn't hurt nearly as much.
- I eat what I want and I want what I eat (but understand that what I want to eat has changed).

- That said, no food is "off limits" and eating sugar/carbs does not "set me off."
- I take a few supplements, but no prescriptions (except bioidentical progesterone cream and a temporary natural thyroid medication. Once my body is working optimally, I won't need this).
- I am more content and confident.
- I trust myself and my body to let me know when I am hungry and when I am satisfied.
- I do not binge.
- I am not hungry all the time.
- I am not guilty, resentful or angry.
- I am love.

At the basis of this balance and healing is the naturopathic approach, which takes into account "mind" and "spirit," in addition to "body." The main difference between it and traditional medicine is a willingness to seek out and address root causes, not just symptoms. It's about getting a body to work as optimally as possible and to look at the reasons why it isn't. It's about coming from a place of love and acceptance, not fear or blame.

I'll give you one example as to how and why my being sick caused me to gain weight, or at the very least, made it difficult for me to lose weight:

Although I had myriad issues, let's look at the Lyme disease (which I am guessing I had for years and which was hiding in my body). My naturopath told me that Lyme neurotoxins block cell receptor sites, so metabolic processes do not work optimally. Hormones (including thyroid), which also help control metabolic processes, can also be affected by Lyme disease.

My thyroid was slightly "off" but still "in range," my adrenal system was "labored," and my stomach was not absorbing necessary vitamins and nutrients. And although it wasn't obvious to me at the time, I didn't feel good.

I didn't notice "not feeling good" right away. There's obvious "not feeling good" like having a bad stomachache or sore throat, and there's subtle "not feeling good" (for example, being slightly tired, having achy joints, or being prone to headaches). It was only when my naturopath spent two hours with me and specifically asked about…everything…that I realized, "hey, maybe I don't feel good."

I had chalked it up to being old and fat…mostly fat. It was a character flaw.

And so what about emotional eating, bingeing, and cravings? How can that be connected? Because my body wasn't able to get the nutrients it needed and I wasn't feeling well in that subtle-yet-acceptable way, I turned to food - especially carbohydrates, which release endorphins (natural tranquilizers) - in order to feel better. That's the coping mechanism I developed as a child. And so one cookie, one small dish of ice cream, one serving of potato chips was never enough…and I was hungry all the time. I felt out of control and pathetic. I was stressed and desperate.

And so the cycle continued.

Although the treatments were unconventional and slower than the traditional approaches, and even though I felt worse before I felt better, I can only come to one conclusion: a holistic approach – which combined my own willingness to accept myself right where I was, naturopathic medicine, and traditional medicine – brought my body into balance.

And as a result, I started losing weight without struggling, without having to "control" myself, without having to count calories, without having lists of "good" and "bad" foods, and without having to exercise to excess. I enjoy all kinds of food. I find pleasure in eating, not guilt. I am relaxed around food. Isn't that the way it's supposed to be?

If you've been struggling for years, can't lose weight – or keep it off – easily and without excessive exercise, chances are something is out of balance. Unfortunately, there is no one-size-fits-all "do this, count that" solution. There is, however, the ability to trust in oneself, and it comes from practicing self-acceptance. It most certainly is a process and it's so much more gratifying and satisfying than coming from a place of fear and self-loathing. I understand that fear-based motivation works initially, but it's not sustainable or healthy in the long run.

Commit to the process of emotional, physical, and spiritual balance and healing. Commit to love, acceptance, enjoyment, pleasure, relaxation, and trust.

Resources...

...some of which are mentioned in the book and some of which are not:

Lynn Gaffin, Open Heart, Open Mind
www.openheart-mind.com
"To try to live with a closed mind is to be blind to the gifts that God, your Higher Power, the Universe, or whatever you choose to call the Infinite, has given you."

Emotional Freedom Technique
www.eftuniverse.com
"The cause of all negative emotions is a disruption in the body's energy system."

Amy G. Martin, Center for Healing Therapies
www.time4healingweb.com
"This is the place where change actually happens."

Dr. Christiane Northrup
www.drnorthrup.com
"An empowering approach to women's health and wellness."

Geneen Roth
www.geneenroth.com
"All that you believe about love, change, joy and possibility is revealed in how, when and what you eat. The world is on your plate."

Dr. David Kessler, The End Of Overeating
www.theendofovereatingbook.com

"...essential for anyone interested in learning more about how corporate greed and human psychology have created a national health crisis."

Charles Seashore
www.american.edu/spa/faculty/cseashore.cfm
"The core of rot."

Thich Nhat Hanh, Savor
www.savorthebook.com
"Mindful eating. Mindful life"

Evelyn Tribole and Elyse Resch, Intuitive Eating
www.intuitiveeating.com
"Creating a healthy relationship with food, mind & body"

Dr. Susan Albers
www.eatingmindfully.com
"How to end mindless eating and enjoy a balanced relationship with food"

American Association of Naturopathic Physicians
www.naturopathic.org
"Naturopathic medicine is based on the belief that the human body has an innate healing ability."

Dr. Brené Brown
www.brenebrown.com
"Authenticity, shame, empathy, vulnerability, courage, compassion, connection."

Martha Beck
www.marthabeck.com
"Find your own peace, purpose, power, and practice."

Acknowledgements

It was Lynn Gaffin, my EFT therapist, who first made me aware of the power of self-acceptance. Thank you Lynn.

It was Amy G. Martin, who developed the Living Lighter class, who was my muse for Parts I and II of this book. Thank you Amy.

It was Dr. John Flaherty and Dr. Jonné Groves who opened my eyes to the power of naturopathic medicine and healing. Thank you Drs. Flaherty and Groves.

It was Elizabeth Irwin, my editor and friend, who took on the task of making sure my words made sense. Thank you Liz.

It was Maria Miranda and Kyisha Bishop, of Miranda Creative, who came up with the concept and design for the cover this book. Thank you Maria and Kyisha.

And then there are the countless friends I have made along the way. Thank you countless friends.

Before these people, there was Lisa Krafick Oorlog, BFF extraordinaire. We've known each other so much longer than we haven't. It's nice to be known the way she knows me. I love you Lisa!

My sister, Holly Brittingham, has been an incredible source of support, wisdom, and love. Her unflagging encouragement is appreciated beyond words. I love you Holly!

And in the beginning, there was my Mom and Dad who loved me first and from whom I continually learn my lessons. Mom, I love you!

My Dad died unexpectedly on New Year's Eve 2010, just before the manuscript for this book went to print. Dad, I know how proud you were of me and you know what? Everything DOES work out the way it is supposed to! Rest in peace, Daddy. I love you!

I'm saving the best for last. He didn't love me first, but he loves me best...and he loved me before I knew how to love myself. He gave me a safe place in which to heal and grow. Thank you dearest, sweetest Tim. If I know what love is, it is because of you. I love you!